Mastering Tai Chi Cane
for Health & Self-Defense

Chen-Style, Yang-Style & Stretch-Massage Forms
Rooted in the Taoist Eight Immortals

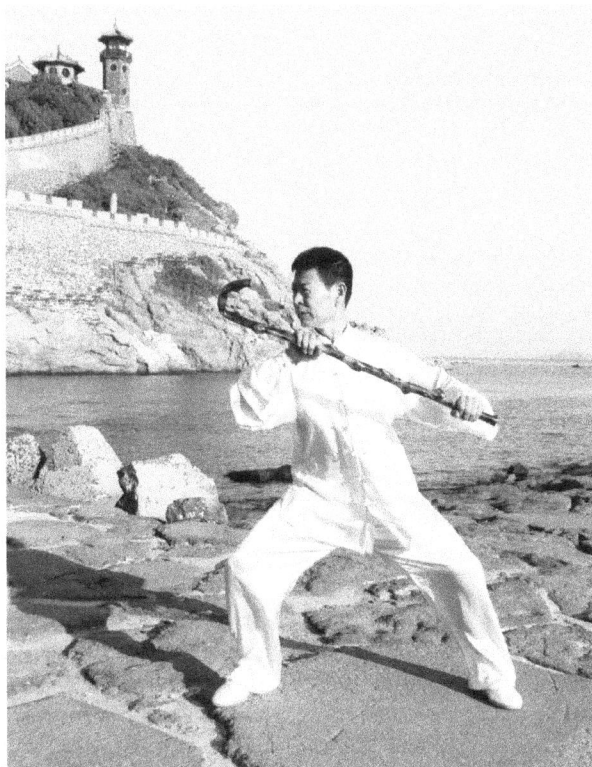

Jesse Tsao, PhD 曹鳳山博士

ISBN: 978-1-7361961-4-4 (Paperback)
ISBN: 978-1-7361961-5-1 (eBook)

The author recommends that you consult your physician regarding the applicability of any recommendations and follow all safety instructions before beginning any exercise program. When participating in any exercise or exercise program, there is the possibility of physical injury. You agree that you do so at your own risk, and are voluntarily participating in these activities.

Chief Editor: Dr. Linda Scott
Book Designer: Heidi Sutherlin
Interior photographs by Jill Whinnery and Tyde Richards
Chinese Calligraphy by Chen Style Tai Chi 11th generation Grandmaster Zhu Tiancai 朱天才
Cover photo: Penglai Temple where the Eight-Immortals legend originated in Dr. Jesse Tsao's hometown, Penglai, China 中國蓬萊閣 courtesy of Dr. Xu Tai-yong 攝影家徐太勇

Contents

Foreword

When my dad first asked me to write this foreword, I turned him down, telling him I couldn't possibly be better qualified than his many accomplished students. I mean, I did learn tai chi from him as a kid, but my adult life has been squarely on the Western allopathic side of medicine. (Please note that the statements here do not reflect my professional opinion as an MD, and the contents of this book should not be considered medical advice, et cetera.) But then he explained he was looking for a more personal perspective, and I couldn't really argue with that since I'd been there the whole way, from when he gave up his solid career as an economist to raise me to the creation of Tai Chi Healthways and sharing the arts of self-healing and self-defense with the wider world.

Many of my childhood hours in brilliant San Diego sunshine were spent behind a video camera capturing my dad practicing his art, framed by crashing waves at the Torrey Pines cliffs. Instead of surfing like a proper coastalite, I was using my fledgling self-taught HTML skills for a more worthy cause than a cute website for our pet parakeets. I still remember the hex code of the horrendous color I chose as the background for my dad's first site, #fde6a8. Designers out there, please forgive me, I was thirteen. But even then I felt that I had to give back in some way, seeing the work ethic that any other child of first-generation immigrants is familiar with. His manifestation of the American Dream involved flying out every week to Arizona for eighteen years to fulfill a continuous contract from the State of Arizona Wellness Office as well as acting as a health education consultant for CIGNA Healthcare using tai chi as a tool for disease prevention that was woven between dozens of group and private classes all over San Diego County.

Perhaps this planted a seed for my eventual career in medicine. Two decades later I became another overeducated millennial still living at his dad's house, getting carried through medical school with the power of home-cooked meals and free laundry. I distinctly remember a humbling moment one sunny afternoon, complaining about my hours on the hospital wards as I watched him recover from a twelve-hour teaching marathon by doing pill bug rolls on a yoga mat, followed by a power nap, only to get up and do it all over again. Talk about leading by example. Before COVID-19 changed the world, he traveled with a frequency that would make my hip Instagrammer friends envious, and still his work ethic bemused us all: "What do you mean you spent four days straight on the workshop and didn't take a single extra hour to sightsee?" Yup, that's just how Master Tsao rolls.

I don't claim mastery or discipleship of any tai chi form, but I did act as an early adopter of sorts for Eight-Immortals Cane, the subject of this book. Per traditional wisdom, my dad made sure to train me properly in a barehand form first, choosing a Chen style fitting of his status as a lineage bearer. Even though I'd spent many hours passively watching him teach while helping him produce videos, it was an entirely different experience to have his focus placed upon me, gently guiding me away from puppeting motions and toward a way of expressing inner intent. It does feel a little magical to have a visualization exercise translate into a much more flowing, effortless movement. While I was doing some research abroad in Liège, he had me hop over to Brussels to perform the Eight-Immortals Cane routine at a costuming ceremony for Manneken Pis, the folkloric symbol of Belgium. It was exactly as surreal as it sounds, being dressed up in the traditional silky garb of an ancient Chinese martial art vis-à-vis a famous statue of a urinating boy wearing the same, followed immediately by attempting to code-switch rapidly between English,

French, and Chinese to dignitaries of The Order of the Friends of Manneken Pis and curious tourists. Apart from being a uniquely memorable experience, I gained a ton of respect for my father for writing and teaching in his second language. It's a testament to decades of experience as a teacher that he can be as precise and creative as he is, improvising with new imagery to help embody the esoteric concepts of "internal practice." Here in this book, you have multiple explanations and photographs for every posture presented to make the occasionally mystical aspects of tai chi practice much more concrete.

With those skills, he's healed thousands of people in his own right before I could spell "ophthalmology." When people ask if I come from a family of doctors, I tell them not exactly, but he beat me to it–he earned his PhD from Shanghai Sports University in 2013 and my MD was awarded in 2017, and thus he's the "OG Dr. Tsao." I have the hands you'd expect for a microsurgeon, sheltered by a cushy lifestyle focused on studying indoors. His hands are big and callused from years of martial arts and manual labor, carrying out the inscrutable will of the Cultural Revolution. Despite my youthful vigor, he can still put me to shame on the proper use of a pickaxe to break earth.

Part of why I like ophthalmology so much is that there's a myriad of skills to learn, from the basics of how to examine an eye all the way to the most advanced intraocular surgery techniques. I wrote my residency applications on this concept of mastery, but maybe I didn't give enough credit to the guy in my house that everyone calls "grandmaster." In this realm of martial arts and Traditional Chinese Medicine, he's become a living treasure. He has dedicated himself utterly to this pursuit, and it is more than a job—his "livelihood" fully became a "way of life." He's attained a near-mythical status with so many as a true master of the craft, but somehow, he's still my funny Asian dad, extolling the virtues of eating two eggs every day and wearing sunscreen, asking what Western medicine has to say about the benefits of being supine by 11:00 p.m. for liver health.

I hope you enjoy your tai chi journey with my dad. I can honestly say that you're in good hands.

Be well,

Jeff Tsao, MD
May 2022

Preface

By far the most frequent message we have received at Tai Chi Healthways is, "I need a book on tai chi cane practice." The contents of this book are my tai chi cane teaching summaries of the last twenty years and the curriculum I created for the Tai Chi Healthways Instructor Program. Tai Chi Healthways is internationally recognized as a leader in tai chi/qigong education and training of the instructors of today and tomorrow to preserve and carry on the classical teachings of the unique Chinese healing art and martial art.

I have taught tai chi cane in Europe since the year 2000. Many tai chi practitioners use these routines and have won gold medals in the European tai chi and martial arts competitions. I have published three instructional DVDs on tai chi cane practice since 2008 (see Video Resources). Recently, more people have expressed a desire for a complete book with demonstration photos for each posture as a teacher's tool or self-study reference to accompany those videos.

Like a cartoon series, intermingled with over three hundred demonstration photos, this book is practical and easy to use and understand. You can practice like a copycat simply imitating a series of photos that show you exactly how to do each move, and then link them together. Plus, detailed instruction and key points for each posture give you pointers for making each move easier and help ensure you're doing them correctly with great form and technique.

Unlike any other manuals, this book provides you with a combination of the cane for fitness, wellness, and self-healing, as well as a martial arts self-defense weapon for all ages, sizes, strengths, or experience and skill level. In a peaceful world, you may never need to use a cane as a weapon for a devastating strike to an opponent, but your years of practice in this system will not be wasted. All your effort spent on the practice will cultivate your vitality for a healthy, long life.

I vividly remembered teaching the cane for stretching and self-massage in Phoenix, Arizona, in the spring of 2015. The course was so popular that all the hooked wooden canes in nearby stores were sold out. Stretching with a cane is excellent for your health. Without the need for a floor mat, these simple yet effective moves can help you limber up for your daily activities, improve your balance to prevent falls, increase your flexibility, loosen up tight muscles, and even help relieve arthritis, back, and knee pain. The cane stretching and self-massage routine is based on Traditional Chinese Medicine (TCM) acupuncture points, tai chi and qigong elements, and is easy to practice anywhere. Each posture has qigong energy circulation benefits and can be customized to your ability ranging from easy to challenging.

The cane stretch and self-massage can be used as a warm-up for natural healing and personal fitness. You can then progress to the Traditional Tai Chi Eight-Immortals Cane Routine I, with a slow and more deliberate tai chi practice to help your body adapt to the moves. Finally, a fast and vigorous practice from Traditional Tai Chi Eight-Immortals Cane Routine II will lead you into the robust leaps and jumps with power strikes. Tai chi cane offers something for everyone.

Jesse Tsao, PhD 曹鳳山博士

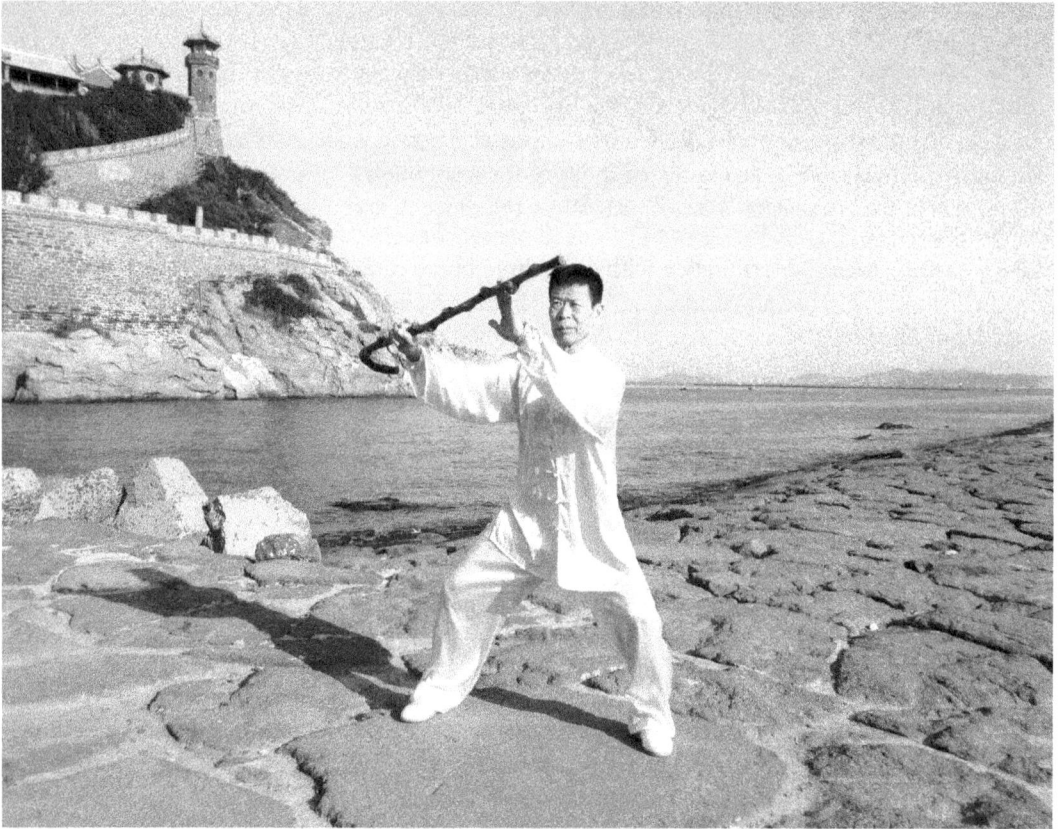

Jesse Tsao practicing Eight-Immortals Tai Chi Cane
Penglai Temple 蓬萊阁 where the Eight Immortals' legend originated

Acknowledgements

I'd like to express my deepest thanks to those masters who guided me in my fifty years of study and research in the arts of self-healing and self-defense. All their collective teachings were merged within this book. I would like to pay my special regards to Jill Whinnery and Tyde Richards who took the interior pictures that greatly enhanced the quality of these posture illustrations.

It is a great honor to have Dr. Linda Scott as the chief editor for this book. As the owner of eFrog Press and as a tai chi student and teacher, she brings a special set of skills to this task. She is a master of words, and her extraordinary language skills were a great contribution to the quality of this book. I also sincerely appreciate the extensive input and editing work from Professor Tom Liu and William Gobron who both practice these cane routines regularly. Gobron, a 4th degree black belt in Uechi Ryu karate, provided valuable suggestions on the cane's martial application.

Words are inadequate in offering my thanks to my Shifu Grandmaster Chen Zhenglei, 陳正雷, 中国當代十大武术名师之一, the 19th generation Chen family and the 11th generation of Chen family tai chi successor, from whom I became a 12th generation of Chen tai chi lineage holder to carry forward the teaching of traditional tai chi methods. Special thanks to Professor Li Deyin 李德印, 北京中国人民大学 who is an icon in Chinese national tai chi coach's training, from whom I learned so much from 1978 to 1987 at Beijing Renmin University. It was a great honor to have Professor Yu Dinghai 虞定海 as my PhD advisor at Shanghai Sport University. Professor Yu is one of the few distinctive experts of nine-duan in both tai chi and qigong fields. In addition to those mentioned above, this book contains the combined knowledge I gathered from many other experts and grandmasters, such as, Chen Xiaowang 陳小旺, Chen Yu 陳瑜, Wu Bin 吳斌, Abraham Liu, Dan Lee, Zang Hongxian 臧洪先, Liu Jishun 劉積順, Su Zifang 蘇自芳, Chen Sitan 陳斯坦, Xie Yelei 謝業雷, and Kong Xiangdong 孔祥東. Any deviations from their teachings are solely my own error.

I would like to extend my deepest gratitude to Grandmaster Zhu Tiancai 朱天才, who encouraged me in the creation and teaching of this Traditional Tai Chi Eight-Immortals Cane, and provided the Chinese calligraphy for the title of this form.

Jesse Tsao, PhD 曹鳳山博士

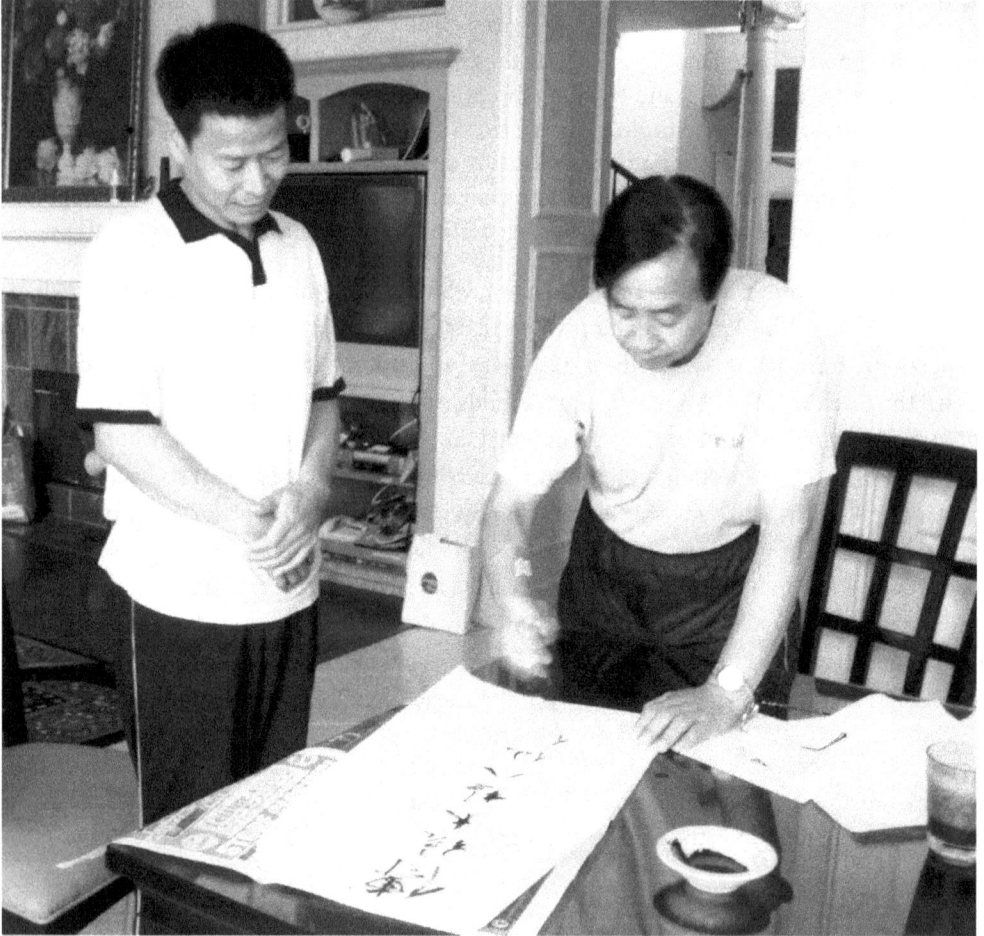

傳統太極八仙杖法

Calligraphy by Grandmaster Zhu Tiancai 朱天才

Chen Style Tai Chi 11th generation

Introduction

Are you worried about your safety after dark in an unsafe neighborhood? Have you considered buying a stun gun or maybe a light dagger? Not necessary. All you need is a cane! A walking cane is commonly seen as a mobility aid for the weak or injured in our daily lives. This innocuous appearance masks its potential as a versatile weapon for self-defense. A cane appears non-threatening with the tip on the ground—which actually provides the opportunity to counterattack with upward-sweeping parries. You can respond instantly to an attacker. While you can't carry traditional weapons in modern life, you can carry a cane or walking stick anywhere in the world including airports, courthouses, and other places that restrict weapons. Martial arts instructors across the world are now teaching cane-fighting techniques. There is a demand for a book to provide a form for instructors and self-study practitioners.

Throughout history the cane has been a self-defense tool in the East and the West. Two thousand years ago, the sage Confucius used his cane to easily block the sword thrusts of the barbarians. In 1912, A.C. Cunningham's manual *The Cane as a Weapon* was published. It is thought to be the only self-defense handbook of its type to be produced in the United States and I have included it here as a supplement. Several European authors produced books and articles on the subject of self-defense with a walking cane in the Victorian era (1837–1901). However, most writings on cane fighting training are tedious with monotonous repetitions of simple parry, jab, thrust, and cut maneuvers.

For tai chi practitioners, the cane is an ideal first weapon. It allows you to further explore tai chi with a blunt object in hand without having to worry about sharp edges. Interwoven in tai chi's circular silk reeling movements, the cane can be used as a shield to block or as a club to strike. Defenses are generally counterattacks to the assailant's weapon or to his weapon-wielding hand. Additional targets for counterattack include the head, face, neck, and midsection. A cane is well-suited for tai chi internal power training because of its explosive smashing, crushing, and wrecking moves. It is especially effective against the bones of the wrist, forearm, shin, and ankle.

Mastering a cane should not be limited to its use as a weapon. This book connects the pleasure of tai chi energy work with cane self-defense applications to make your training an enjoyable art. So, it is not a simple strike and hit motion; it is a course of energy cultivation for your wellness and fitness as well as skills to keep assailants at bay. A cane is an extension of your arm. You will learn to train the extension of your body's energy through your mind and intention to develop the ability to send your internal power through the length of a cane.

More than just a martial arts weapon or mobility aid, the cane has held numerous functions of significance from the ancient Chinese cane dancing to the glamorous canes for the dapper gentlemen of the 20s. Canes are embedded in the culture of almost every country around the globe. Based on my PhD research and more than twenty years of teaching experience, I will guide you along an easily accessible route to complete mastery of the cane.

I was born in Penglai, on the Shandong Peninsula of China (中国蓬莱). Penglai is a coastal town known as the "Fairyland on Earth" where the legendary Eight Immortals are believed to have dwelled and practiced their immortality. I was exposed to the rich Taoist culture. I grew up with the practice of the Taoist Eight Immortals martial arts, as well as tai chi.

According to Chinese mythology, the Eight Immortals lived in the middle of the Bohai Sea (渤海) on Mount Penglai which was situated on a beautiful, paradise-like island. The Eight Immortals are a group of ancient, legendary heroes who fight for justice and vanquish evil. Their stories have been part of Chinese oral history long before they were recorded in the works of writers of various dynasties. They represent separately the male, the female, the old, the young, the rich, the noble, the poor, and the humble. Their stories encourage people to work hard on their practice to achieve longevity.

One story is called "The Eight Immortals Crossing the Sea from the Taoist Penglai Temple (八仙過海)." The legend is about the Immortals on a journey to attend the conference of the Magical Peach at the Celestial Heaven (蟠桃會). Instead of going across the sea by floating on their clouds—the Immortals' way of transportation—their leader, Lu Dongbin, suggested that they use their magical power to cross. Stemming from this story is a Chinese proverb: "The Eight Immortals cross the sea, each reveals their divine power (八仙過海，各显其能)."
Each Immortal's power could be transferred to a power tool, a kind of talisman associated with a certain meaning that can give life or destroy evil.

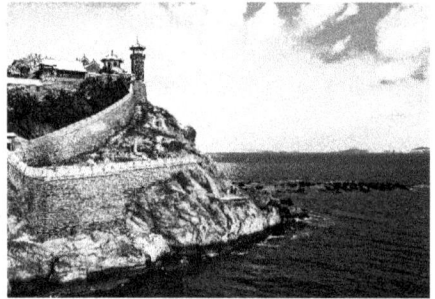

There are many martial art routines named after the Immortals' stories, such as the Eight-Immortals Sword, Eight-Immortals Fist, Eight-Immortals Fan, and Eight-Immortals Flute. The Traditional Tai Chi Eight-Immortals Cane is one of the routines I created, named after Tieguai Li (鐵枴李), the Iron-Crutch Li. He is always depicted as a beggar with a crutch. Legend explains his lame state as follows: His spirit would frequently leave his body briefly to wander in the celestial regions. His body on earth is in the charge of his disciple. On one occasion, Li asked his disciple to watch over his physical body for seven days and prevent its destruction by animals, insects, and other spirits. He told his disciple to burn his body after seven days if he had not returned by then. After only six days the disciple learned that his own mother was dying, so he burned Li's body and went to his mother's bedside. Li returned on the seventh day and could not find his body, so he entered the corpse of a lame beggar who had just died. He blew water on the beggar's bamboo staff and changed it into an iron crutch. He also carries a pilgrim's bottle-gourd. The gourd symbolizes longevity and the ability to ward off evil and to help the needy. He is well-known to the poor, sick, and needy for his reputation for benevolence.

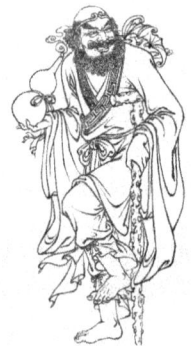

Here are short stories of the other Immortals:

Lu Dongbin was one of the most popular of the Eight Immortals and was considered to be the leader. Lu usually depicted holding a Taoist flybrush in his right hand and a sword slung over his back. He used this sword to slay dragons and demons. Carrying the sword on his back and living in moderation meant that he was always vigilant to not stray from the middle path. He always used the sword to cleave away any temptations to stray. In the Eight-Immortals Sword, this means that there are no excesses or insufficiencies and every technique adheres to the middle or balanced path.

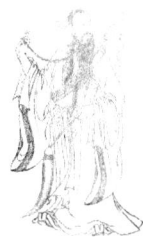

Zhang Guolao was a recluse who had supernatural powers. He could make himself invisible. It is said that he enjoyed traveling at least a thousand miles a day on the back of his trusty white mule facing backward, and thus is often depicted riding a mule in this manner. Upon reaching his destination, he collapsed the mule and folded it like a piece of paper and stored it in his pocket. When ready to travel again he would take it out, and moisten it with water to change it back into a mule. His emblem is a bamboo instrument that is struck with two rods and a tube containing wands or "phoenix feathers" with which he can foretell fortunes and misfortunes. He is known to help souls reincarnate.

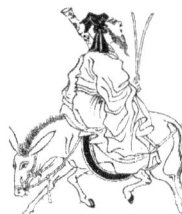

Zhong Lichuan was an army general. After meeting an old man who taught him about Taoism, he left government service and went to the mountains becoming a wanderer and a beggar. One day his meditation chamber was filled with rainbow clouds and celestial music. A crane arrived and carried him on its back into the regions of immortality. He is portrayed as bearded and thinly clad. His hair is gathered in two coils on the side of his head. His symbol is a fan, which he uses to revive and reincarnate the souls of the departed. Sometimes he also holds a peach.

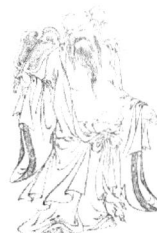

Tsao Guojiu was not a popular Immortal because he was so fierce. It was said that he was a member of the Imperial Court and was a very dangerous person to tangle with. He is feared greatly by both ghosts and goddesses wherever he goes. He gave away all his wealth to the poor and went into the mountains to seek the Tao. After some time, he harmonized his mind, body, and spirit until he could easily transform himself into the Tao. One day while roaming about his mountain realm he met two of the eight Immortals, Zhong Lichuan and Lu Dongbin. Lu asked him, "What are you doing?" He replied, "I am nurturing the Tao and studying the Way." Asked where the Tao was, Tsao pointed to heaven. Asked where heaven was, he pointed to his heart. Zhong beamed and said, "The heart is heaven and heaven is the Tao. You indeed found the truth and the Way. You understand the origin of things." They invited him to travel with other Immortals. His symbol is the castanets, which were made from the court tablet. He played in a soothing and relaxing rhythm to facilitate meditation and journeying throughout the universe. He is mounted upon a horse whose spirit may have helped him unveil the secrets of the Tao and immortality.

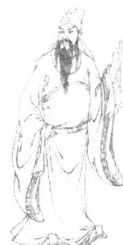

Han Xiangzi was a nephew of the great Tang poet and scholar, Han Yu. It is believed that he could make flowers grow and blossom instantly. His emblem is the flute and he is the patron saint of musicians. He is depicted as very young and it is said that he did not like to use his sword. But when he did use his sword, no one could escape. He was initiated into the secrets of Taoism by fellow Immortal Lu Dongbin while still a teenager and quickly became absorbed in the practice of internal alchemy. It is also said that Han traveled the countryside playing his flute and attracting birds and beasts of prey with the beautiful sound.

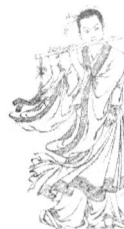

He Xiangu became an immortal at age fourteen after meeting fellow Immortal Lu Dongbin, who taught her internal alchemy and gave her a precious, rare Peach of Immortality. Soon after eating the peach, she was able to journey in her spirit body to pay homage to the Great Taoist Goddess of Immortality. She was able to cease her menstruation and conserve her life force energy. She also gained the ability to nourish herself by feeding only upon sweet, heavenly dew and the omnipresent Chi. She spent her youth telling fortunes, flying, and floating from mountain peak to mountain peak collecting herbs for her mother and the poor. She ignored the royal command and instead ascended to heaven in full daylight, disappearing from the earth. She is usually depicted holding a magic lotus blossom, the flower of openheartedness and divine brilliance, which symbolizes her power and purity.

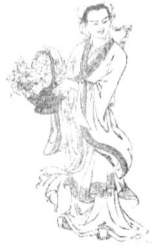

Lan Caihe, the particular Immortal, is sometimes depicted as a female and sometimes as a male, the Immortal Hermaphrodite. He/she was an entertainer and like some ancient shamans wore women's sexually ambiguous clothing and makeup. A street singer and a beggar, he gave away his money to the poor. Always dancing and singing, he walked about with one bare foot, followed by crowds who thought he was crazy. In winter he would sleep soundly in the snow with steam rising from his body—a sure sign that he had mastered the techniques of internal alchemy. One evening, after singing and entertaining, he left a tavern and mounted a crane that had descended amidst the sounds of a celestial chorus. The crane gracefully carried him into the sky before an astounded crowd. His symbol is a basket of flowers, plants, and branches from trees associated with longevity, such as chrysanthemum, peach blossom, and sprigs of pine and bamboo. He is mounted on an elephant, a symbol of wisdom, strength, and prudence.

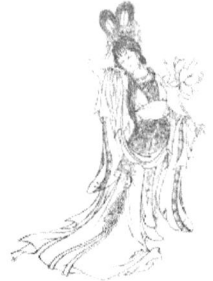

It has been my longtime desire to share the arts I have learned and benefited from to honor my hometown's culture. I do not want the teachings of the masters of my hometown to be lost. Tai chi and the Taoist practice saved my health. Malnutrition from early childhood caused my sickness. I was born during the Great Chinese Famine (三年自然灾害大饥荒), "three years of great famine"), a period between 1959 and 1961. Some scholars have also included the years 1958 and 1962. This famine is widely regarded as one of the greatest disasters in human history. When I was seven years old, congenital energy insufficiency hindered my normal development. My mother obtained a special herbal medicine but the horrible taste resulting from concentrating the essence from the woody plant's roots and bark made me vomit. So, my Traditional Chinese Medicine (TCM) doctor suggested that my mother seek the help of Taoist practice. In TCM, a boy's development follows an eight-year cycle (a girl's development follows a seven-year cycle). To be healthy, a boy's kidney energy needs to be flourishing by the age of eight (丈夫八岁·肾气实). I started my Taoist energy practice to improve my health. I was taught how to take the essence from nature through breathing (食气法), and how to use the Five Animal Frolics to release sickness and gather universal energy (五禽戏导引功法). Thankfully, the Taoist practices worked well for me, and I was filled with vital energy by the age of sixteen. In this book, I share the combined knowledge of more than fifty years of traditional training and my formal academic education including a PhD in Traditional Chinese Martial Arts Education from the Shanghai University of Sport.

This book is divided into three parts and each focuses on one of the three cane routines I have created. Part 1 is a routine based on the Taoist Eight-Immortals short stick martial function, which itself is based on the traditional Yang-style tai chi postures with the characteristic softer flow and circular movements. Part 2 is a routine mixed with the Eight-Immortals short stick self-defense and traditional Chen-style tai chi cannon fist postures characterized by powerful movements and explosive strikes. Part 3 introduces the Tai Chi Qigong Cane Stretch and Self-Massage, which is an easy and effective preventative and self-healing practice. It is a combination of tai chi, qigong, and TCM energy points that eliminate your body's blockages to let energy flow, flushing out stress and cleaning out stagnation and toxins.

Before you start to learn the postures and begin practicing, you should be equipped with some fundamental knowledge.

Footwork and Stances

There are seven major stances in the routines: horseback riding stance, bow stance, empty stance, rooster stance, low stance (snake creeps down), crossing stance, and resting stance. You do not need to pose the stances perfectly. But you do need to be comfortable and relaxed, yet, at the same time, alert and ready for movement. For the full development of the cane as a weapon of defense and attack, it is necessary to be able to quickly change the position of the body without loss of balance or control. This change is accomplished by the movement of your feet stepping forward, backward, to the right, or to the left side. Footwork serves your torso's motion (步随身换). Pay attention to the direction of your toes. Your feet may quickly change from one to the other by reversing the direction your toes are pointing.

- Horseback riding stance
- Bow stance
- Empty stance
- Rooster stance

- Low stance (or half-low stance)
- Crossing stance
- Resting stance

Tai chi stances can be performed at three different heights: high, medium, and low. The height depends on your flexibility and how warmed up you are. Do not try a low stance until you have warmed up your body. Start in a high stance, and then over time lower your stance and continue to practice.

1. Horseback riding stance 马步

Stand with your feet about double shoulder-width apart, feet parallel to one another, and squat down. Evenly distribute your weight, fifty percent on each leg. Keep your head suspended and pelvis down, chest relaxed, and back full. There should not be more tension in your knees than in your hips. Sink your hips toward your heels to prevent knees bending over your toes. The overall sensation is that your upper body is light and your lower body is heavy. Squat as low as you can sustain in a relaxed way throughout this stance practice.

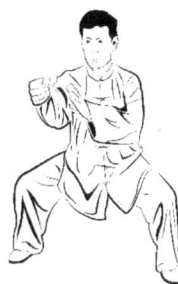

Horseback riding stance is regarded as a bitter training method because it is sometimes used by a teacher to test the sincerity and obedience of a potential disciple. Your squat can be as low as bringing the thighs parallel to the ground. This means the inguinal creases, the angle of your stomach to thigh, is almost ninety degrees. Horseback riding stance builds a strong foundation of leg strength and balance. It is one of the stances that does not have a left and right form, as you distribute your body's weight equally between each foot and leg. It is called the mother stance because the other stances—with various weight distributions, angles of feet, and leg twists—are created from the horseback riding stance.

2. Bow stance 弓步

Bow stance is the basic, forward-weighted stance used in all martial arts. Seventy percent of the weight should be on the forward leg and thirty percent on the rear. In tai chi practice, do not completely straighten the rear leg. Instead, open rear leg inguinal crease with knee pointed out slightly, and the flexed knees will provide stability and agility. Bring the front thigh as close to parallel to the ground as you are able, but your front knee should not be extended forward over the toes. Develop your lower stance by sliding your back foot out farther with the spine aligned to allow your body to sink.

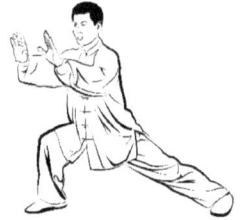

The bow stance is the classic stance for the delivery of power. It appears frequently throughout tai chi forms. You need to properly position your feet to ensure good balance. It is particularly important not to cross the legs; keep one foot on either side of your centerline for better balance. The toes of the back foot should be turned out at a forty-five to seventy degree angle. This stance is also called a mountain climbing stance.

3. Empty stance (commonly called cat stance) 虚步

In an empty stance, most of your weight is on the rear leg with the toes or heel of the front foot lightly touching the ground. The empty stance has the greatest potential for quick movement, since it allows for a kick or step in any direction without needing to transfer your weight to move. This stance is also called cat stance as it displays the spirit of an alert cat ready to react agiley. Start this stance standing high and as your legs become stronger, drop the stance lower and lower while holding it for longer periods of time. Drop the hip of your weighted leg toward the heel to prevent injuring your knee.

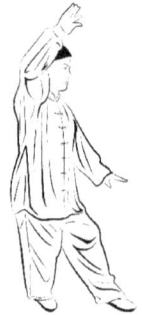

Empty stance is a good practice to improve your leg's bone density. Your body weight shifting from two legs to one leg can be extremely beneficial for preventing bone loss in older adults. "Performing weight-bearing and resistance training exercises can help increase bone formation during bone growth and protect bone health in older adults, including those with low bone density." (Franziska Spritzler, RD, CDE, "10 Natural Ways to Build Healthy Bones," *Healthline*, August 12, 2019, https://www.healthline.com/nutrition/build-healthy-bones)

4. Rooster stance 金鸡独立式

The rooster stance is a one-legged stance. Put all your weight on one foot, and lift the knee of the unweighted leg high. The single-leg stance promotes balance and stability as well as leg strength. It is also the foundational training for kicks in tai chi practice. Tai chi practice is slow-motion in training. To perform any kick in slow-motion, single-leg stability and strength is required to raise up the knee of the kicking leg to waist height before extending into a slow-motion kick. Be sure to line up your head, pelvis, and foot in a muscle-relaxed, vertical alignment.

Rooster stance is a popular practice in China. It is believed, based on TCM theory, that when one foot supports the body's weight, the blood and energy

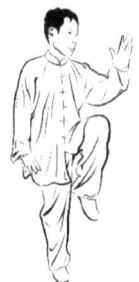

flow circulates through the six meridian channels reaching to your foot more effectively. The improved energy circulation will balance the blood pressure and improve the function of multiple inner organs, as well as prevent insomnia.

5. Low stance 仆步

Sink slowly onto one crouched leg while you slide the other foot along the ground until that leg is straight (with the knee unlocked). Both feet must be flat on the ground. The back is straight and almost upright. Your head faces the stretched leg. If you cannot crouch completely down without lifting a heel off the floor or bending your torso forward, only go halfway down or as low as you are able to maintain good, comfortable torso posture. Bring the rear thigh as close to your calf as you are able.

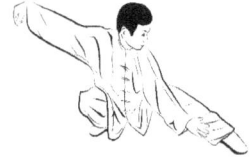

The low stance stretches the inner leg muscles of that extended leg and strengthens the rear leg muscles. It trains your mobility in a lower position, which gives you the ability to change levels from a high stance to a medium or low stance with ease. It helps your footwork become more agile.

6. Cross stance 叉步

In cross stance, one leg is crossed behind the other as when you step sideways or are preparing for a spin. From a shoulder-width stance, bend both knees and hips slightly, then cross one leg behind and extend it as far as you can in a stretch. The supporting front leg will bend lower at hip and knee as close to ninety degrees as comfortably possible. Start at a comfortable height, and slowly develop the lower-level stretch and leg strength. Alternate the legs to train both evenly. This stance is a good practice to train the waist-turning flexibility.

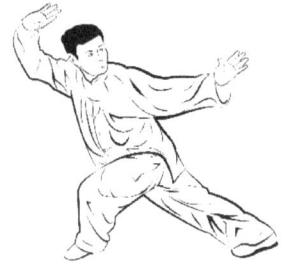

7. Resting stance 歇步

Squat down with one knee under the other. The heel of the lower leg is off the ground. Your buttocks should rest on the lower calf and the back of the heel but your weight is mainly on the front leg. Keeping your knees lined up with the direction of your toes will prevent hurting your knees. Keep your upper body vertical and your back totally extended. Don't lean forward at all. Keep your head up and look horizontally. Alternate the legs to train both evenly. This stance is a good practice to prevent sciatic pain.

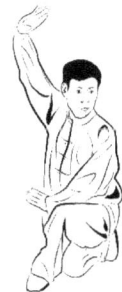

Holding the Cane

Usually, you hold the cane in one hand and sometimes you grasp the cane in both hands. When holding with a single hand, grasp the cane at a distance of six to eight inches from the handle hook/butt. This position gives a balance that permits very quick motions and allows both the tip point and the butt/hook to be brought into use. The position of your thumb changes instantly. For close direction and control, your thumb may be extended along the cane; for free-swinging cuts, your thumb may be grasped around the cane. The knuckles (or the palm) may be turned up, down, or to either side. Your grasp should be sufficiently firm to prevent the cane from slipping through or being knocked from your hand.

A perfect cane for all-purpose practice is a natural wood one with a rounded hook. An ideal length is measured from the floor to the height of your hip socket and may be up to your belly button, on average 36–42 inches long and one inch in diameter. The weight may range from one to two pounds depending on the type of wood. The cane may also have multiple natural knots, like the cane pictured here, which are ideal for massage. The hook end is called the butt or the handle, and the tip end of the cane is called the tail or tip.

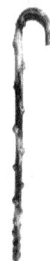

Parry and Counter Blow

Taoist Eight-Immortals cane self-defense primarily uses parry (*lan-jie* 拦截) and counter blow. When the attack is made with a knife or other weapon, parry is the best to deflect sideways with your knuckles turned in the direction of the parry. At the same time, your counter blow should be directed against the assailant's hand or forearm.

Jab and Thrust

The jab (*chuo* 戳) and thrust (*ci* 刺) are among the most effective blows that can be given with a cane as they are concentrated and the force will penetrate the attacker's body. Jab is a short stabbing blow given with either the tip point or the butt of the cane. Normally it is preceded by a small drawing back of the hand to impart more force. The jab is one of the quickest attacks with a cane. The tip-point jab is best made with your thumb along the cane; the hook/butt-jab may be made with your thumb around the cane and is mostly used on a large target area, such as the chest. The thrust is a stabbing blow and differs from the jab in that it is delivered over a longer distance with full extension of your arm and with the weight of your body behind the blow.

Cut and Chop

To execute a cut (*zhan-kan* 斩砍), focus on a certain point where the full force of the blow will be delivered. The force should be cumulative up to the objective point and should cease as soon as possible after this is reached. There are a variety of cuts. Snap cut is short and quick and initiates most of the motion and force from the wrist. Half-arm cut starts from your elbow and includes a wrist snap. The preliminary position will start from your shoulder, but when the cut is delivered it will be mainly from your elbow. Full-arm cut is delivered from your shoulder and includes more or less elbow and wrist motion. Swinging or sweep cut is made in a horizontal plane over a long arc and may be continued back and forth. Its principal use is for keeping the distance open. Sometimes a swinging cut can be used vertically on the side of your body. Down cut is very strong and hard and is also called chop or hack. Other categories are based on direction. Upper cut is made from downward to upward. It may not be strong, but the upper cut is valuable as there are no preliminary indications so it is hard to avoid. Right cut or left cut, either high or low, requires more or less preparation in the opposite direction with the knuckles of the hand holding the cane turned in the direction of the blow. Diagonal cut travels in an angular direction from the vertical or horizontal and may be upward or downward, right or left. Circular cut moves in full, continuous swings. The first swing is away from the object and the continuation is toward the object. Backhanded cut (*liao* 撩) is made with the knuckles turned away from the direction of the blow. The upper and left cuts are most successfully made backhanded.

Tai Chi's Peng-Lu-Ji-An 掤挒擠按 as the Adhesive

Tai chi's circular, soft energy serves as the adhesive to the cane's striking motions. Any posture's movement can be interpreted as these four primary tai chi energies: *peng-lu-ji-an.*

Peng *(掤勁)* is an energy of ward off, rise up and support, expand, brace, curved barrier, or buffer zone. Forming energy circles to meet and support an incoming force is the peng's main function. It is the essential energy; all others are a manifestation of peng. Without peng, no further jins will emerge.

Lu *(挒勁)* is an energy of roll back, waist turning, deflect, redirect, neutralize, avert, fend off to redirect incoming force. Before rolling back, you must deliberately initiate using ward-off energy.

Ji *(擠勁)* is a press, squeeze, extend, and concentrated energy. Squeeze in with the body, and send your body into a dominant position.

An *(按勁)* is an energy of seal, constraint with pressure, control and cover, push and drive away. There must be coordination between your hands and feet, and the push power is from your waist and legs combined with increased intention.

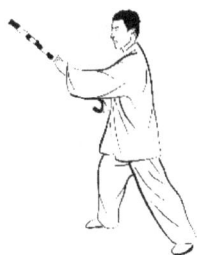 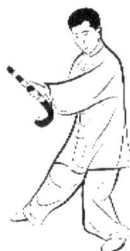 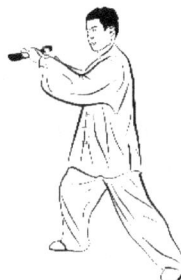 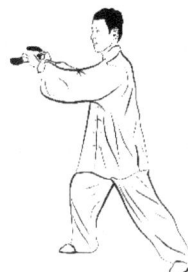

1. Ward Off   **2. Rollback**   **3. Press**   **4. Push/Pouncing**

1. Ward Off

Step into a bow stance with your right foot in front, and at the same time swing the cane in front of your chest diagonally with your left palm gently touching the middle part of the cane. Imagine the cane length is the extension of your right forearm. With the tail of the cane, intercept your attacker's knife or club and adhere to it. Keep the body of your cane covering your front diagonally, with the hook in front of your right hip, the middle part of the cane in front of your left shoulder, and the tail of the cane head high and lined up with your left ear. This posture is derived from the barehand tai chi ward-off posture and forms a solid protection for the upper part of your body (Figure 1).

2. Rollback

Turn your torso a little toward your left and shift weight back to your left foot; at the same time turn the tip of your cane in a small counterclockwise circle by flipping your right palm to face downward while holding the cane to redirect an attack sliding toward your left side. Don't miss the small turning at the tip of the cane. It is important to smoothly coil your cane from the left side to the right side of the attacker's weapon in order to deflect it to the outside of your body. This flipping of the right palm is the same as your barehand form. Turning your torso to the left side is also important to guide the attacker's weapon away from you (Figure 2).

3. Press

To press, shift weight forward and press the cane forward with both hands. The horizontal cane serves the same role as your forearms in the barehand form's press. This is the motion to occupy the battlefield and to not give the attacker any space to operate his weapon. The best result is to seal his weapon to his torso (Figure 3).

4. Push/Pouncing

Drop the cane a little with a small step back to give yourself a crouching pose to gather the earth's energy. Next, follow up with a big forward blow like a powerful tiger pouncing (Figure 4).

Adhere to Tai Chi's Basic Aspects for Energy Cultivation

Keep the crown of your head (百会) lifting upward while your jaw relaxes downward with the tip of your tongue resting on the area behind your front upper teeth (搭鹊桥), which bridges the *yang* energy on your body's back and *yin* energy on the front of your body in the process of transforming into a unified force. Root your feet into the ground for better central equilibrium with the heels and the balls of the front of the feet (*yong-quan* 涌泉穴) connecting with the earth's energy. Sink to establish the foundation and stability before you rise. Yin gives birth to yang. Yin and yang alternate and harmonize (阴阳互变) in any move simultaneously. Drop your shoulders and sense the roundness and fullness of your upper back. Unlock your hips and knees to store strength as if a bow is about to release an arrow.

The Facing Direction

If possible, face the south to start each form with your left side to the east and your right side to the west. Your front torso belongs to yin (阴) and your back belongs to yang (阳). Traditionally, tai chi is practiced outdoors, so the direction you face will help you harmonize your body with nature for better energy exchange with the universe. The south is yang and the north is yin. The directions in this book will be based on the assumption that you began the form facing south.

In the following pages, I will show you how to master the cane through tai chi practice. I'll walk you through step by step with many photographs to demonstrate each pose in detail. The cane is not just a mobility aid. The cane is an auxiliary training tool to improve your balance, agility, and vitality for your lifetime.

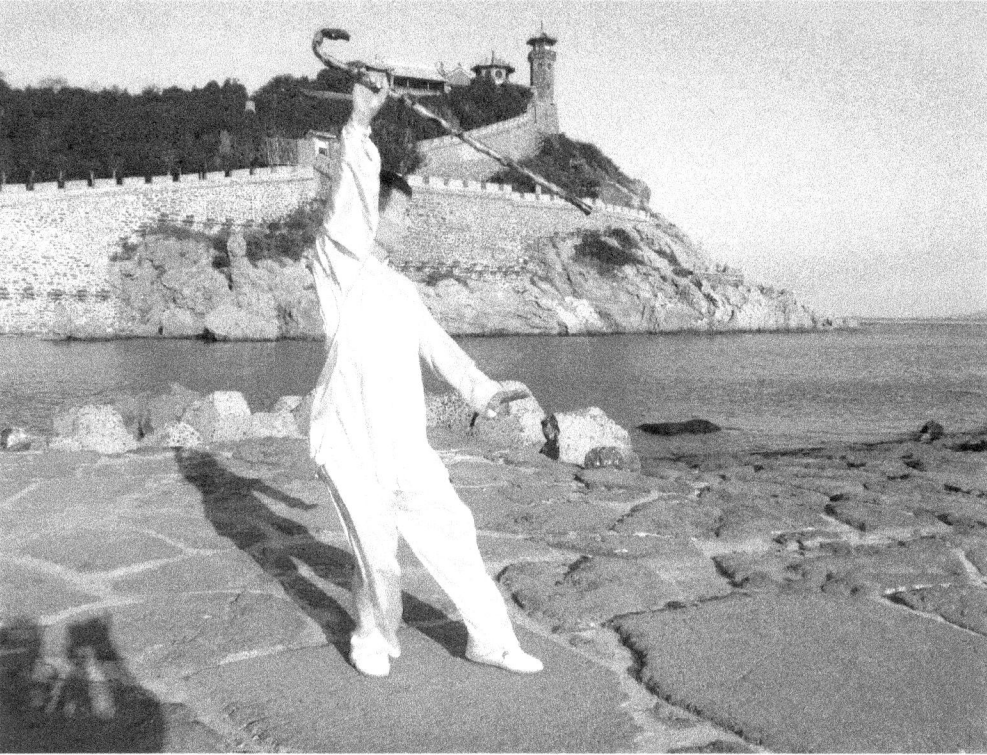

白鹤亮翅

White Crane
Spreads Wings

Part 1
Traditional Tai Chi Eight-Immortals Cane - Routine 1

This routine is based on the characteristics of Yang-style tai chi postures with the traditional Taoist "Eight Immortals" cane/stick martial function. It is fun for any age or skill level to learn. Yang style is the most popular tai chi style, widely practiced around the globe. When I choreographed this routine, I emphasized the slow, even, gentle, and large movements. If you practice the traditional Yang tai chi, you will naturally adapt to the cane play.

Section 1

Posture 1: Opening Form 太極起勢

Movement 1

Stand relaxed with feet parallel and step out with your left foot, shoulder-width apart. Loosen your waist and unlock your hips to lower your center of gravity. Find your central equilibrium by containing your chest and lifting your spine as if an intangible energy rope were pulling up the crown of your head. Imagine there is a central axis passing through your torso from head to tailbone. Stay in this pose for a moment until you feel your spine elongate and the spaces between your vertebrae open. The cane is at the side of your right leg, near the right foot. Calm your mind and settle your breath down deep into the lower abdomen (Photo 1-1).

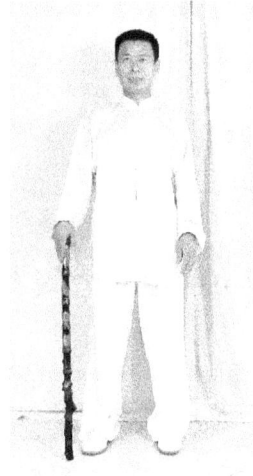

Photo 1-1

Movement 2

Sink your left hip a little more and turn your torso to your right, chest facing the southwest corner. At the same time, sink your shoulders and circle your left hand up in front of your chest to chin height with palm facing toward your chest. Feel the peng (ward off) energy as you maintain a space between your left arm and your chest (Photo 1-2).

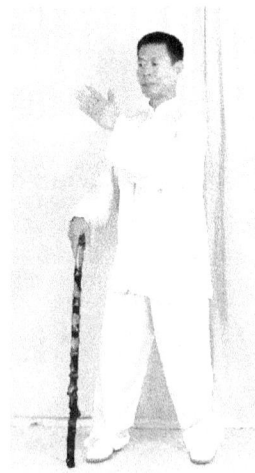

Photo 1-2

Movement 3

Turn your torso to the left and move your left palm outward in an upper curve toward the southeast front corner. At the same time, turn the left palm facing outward, and let your eyes follow your left hand (Photo 1-3).

Movement 4

Circle your left palm down and return it to the left side of your belly. Sink both hips a little more by bending both knees slightly and settle down your *dantian* (the center of your lower abdomen) with a deep exhale. You should feel your crotch (the space between your inner thighs) round like an arched stone bridge and a gentle outward pressure on your inner thighs. The ward-off energy of your pelvis enables you to hold your torso in a stable position (Photo 1-4).

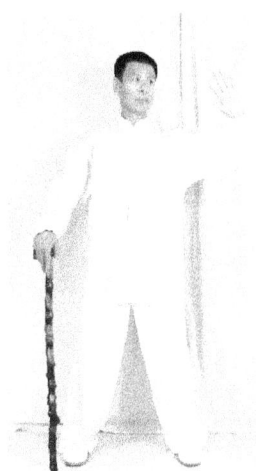

Photo 1-3

Key Points

1) If possible, face the south to start the form with your left side to the east and your right side to the west. The directions that follow assume you began the form facing to the south.

2) The preparation is to relax the mind and body to allow your inner energy to circulate without blockage.

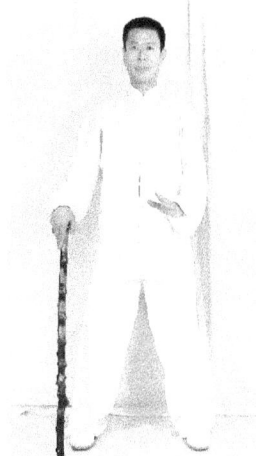

Photo 1-4

3) Sink your left hip to get the earth's rebound energy for your dantian rotation to give birth to the silk reeling of your left hand. Let your torso motion lead your arm and hand.

4) Your left hand traces the curves of the tai chi symbol circling up in front of your chest, curving down along the s-pattern, and circling up to take over the cane.

5) At the end, unlock and sink your hips to round your crotch to be ready for the next move.

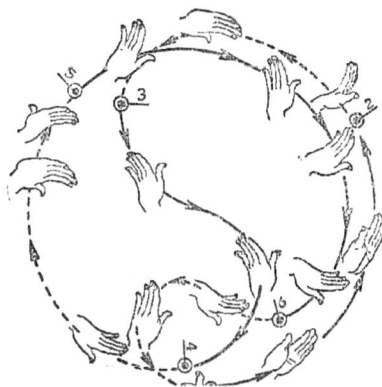

Posture 2: Strike the Gong 撞锤势

Movement 1

Slide your right hand down from the top of the cane handle-hook, about five to six inches from the end. Turn your torso slightly to your left front southeast corner and swing the cane up in front of your body. Grasp the lower part (tail) of the cane with your left hand. Use your arms to position the cane in front of your chest while keeping your elbows unlocked and your shoulders relaxed (not raised). Maintain the sinking of your hips and gently push your lower back backward to support the cane's forward extension in a bracing position to guard your left front (Photo 2-1).

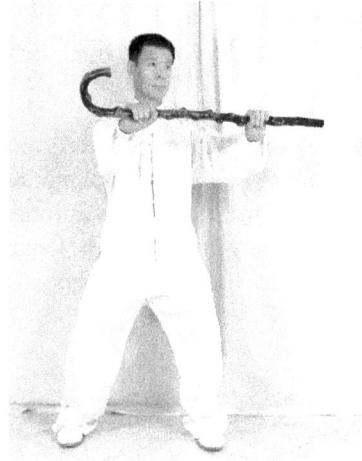

Movement 2

Shift weight to your left heel and slightly turn your right heel toward your right front southwest corner to open your right hip as you turn your torso to the right. At the same time, twist the cane in a clockwise direction with the tip pointed slightly upward as if you are redirecting an incoming weapon targeting your face. Power the cane from your torso's turning energy. Your arms adapt to the torso's motion by pulling the cane handle toward your right rib side and pushing the left hand end of the cane out with the left palm open behind the cane. Your left hand is protected from your opponent's weapon by the cane. This motion is called lu, the roll-back in tai chi terms (Photo 2-2).

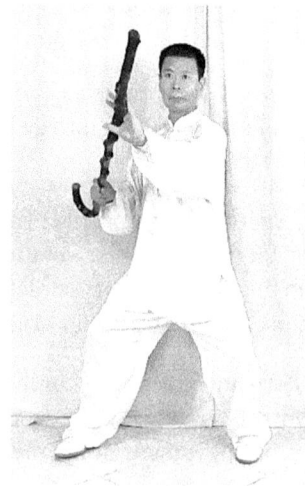

Photo 2-1

Photo 2-2

Movement 3

Shift weight to your right foot, and draw your left foot in and place it a half-step distance in front of your right foot. At the same time, lower the cane to waist level and draw it against your right rib side. In this gathering in and storing up energy pose, you are like a crouching tiger waiting for the opportunity to pounce upon its prey (Photo 2-3).

Movement 4

Sink your right hip and use the rebound energy from the earth to power the stepping of your left foot forward, and thrust the cane tip to the front at heart level. Optionally, leap with your left foot and follow up with your right to create the momentum for the strike (Photo 2-4).

Key Points

1) Make sure to move the cane with your torso, not your arms. The energy travels from your feet through your legs to your torso.

2) This sequence is a typical tai chi application: ward off, roll back, press, and push (peng-lu-ji-an). You use the cane as your arm's extension to make contact with your opponent's weapon, adhere to it with the ward-off energy, then use your torso's move to redirect the incoming force sideways, followed by pressing in your body to seal the opponent's weapon and strike him back.

3) The forward strike is powered by your body's movement, especially your back right foot and left hand connection to guide the power to the tip of the cane.

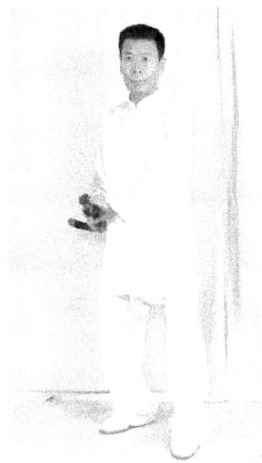

Photo 2-3

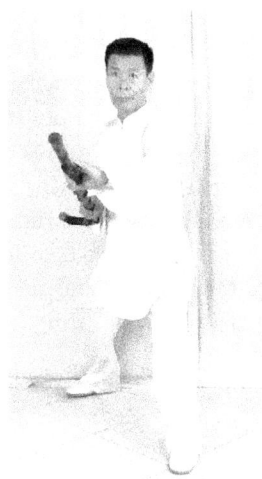

Photo 2-4

Posture 3: Paddle Across the Ocean 八仙過海

Movement 1

Tilt the cane tip up and turn it clockwise in an upward curve toward your right front corner (southwest) as if to deflect a weapon attacking your face. Initiate the cane's movement from the turning of your torso. Your head moves slightly to your left side while the cane tip parries to the right front (Photo 3-1).

Movement 2

Circle the cane tip in a downward curve in front of your knee from the right side to your left hip. Shift weight back to your right foot and withdraw the left foot halfway back with toes touching the floor (heel a few inches off the floor). This is called a left empty stance. At the same time, pull the cane tip back toward your torso, slide your left hand down, and push the cane handle forward with your right palm while sliding your right palm down to leave enough length at the cane handle end for the forward ward off to defend your front high position (Photo 3-2).

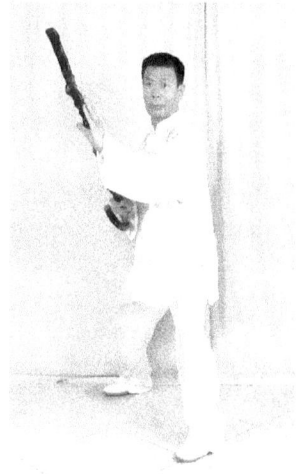

Photo 3-1

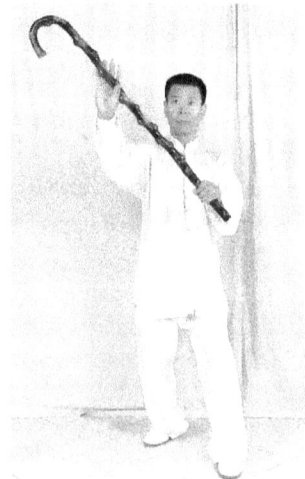

Photo 3-2

Movement 3

Step your left foot to the left front corner (southeast) and bend your left knee to shift weight onto your left foot while pulling the cane handle back toward your right ribs. At the same time, push the cane tail side from your left ribs toward your right front upper corner (southeast) as if you were warding off a weapon targeting your head. The cane's motion is driven by your torso's turning to the right. While doing so, slide both of your hands down six to eight inches toward the cane handle (Photo 3-3).

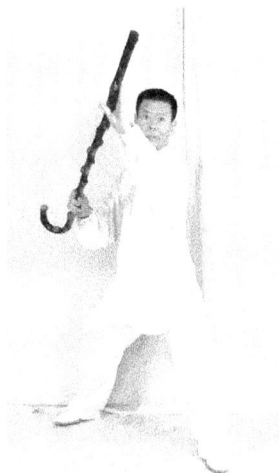

Movement 4

Push the cane to the right front (southwest) corner as your right arm extends without locking up the right elbow. At the same time, ward off your left palm to the left front (southeast) corner with the left arm curved in a half-moon shape. Your eyes look at the middle of the cane (Photo 3-4).

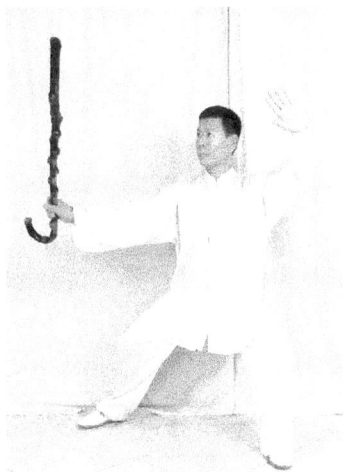

Key Points

1) Remember, the turning of the body initiates the motion of the arms, and the cane is an extension of your arms.

2) Keep your torso erect, drop your shoulders, and keep your elbows down.

3) Adjust your hand position on the cane, alternately grasping and opening your fingers.

Photo 3-3

Photo 3-4

Posture 4: Grasp Bird's Tail 揽雀尾

Movement 1

Pull your right foot back toward your left foot with the right toes touching the floor. At the same time, move the cane in a downward curve as if to deflect an incoming weapon targeting your left side. Close your left hand in with a palm press on the cane to reinforce the roll back action (Photo 4-1).

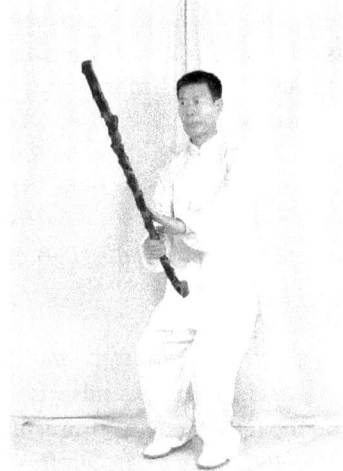

Photo 4-1

Movement 2

Step your right foot to your right side (the west) and shift weight to your right leg to form a bow stance. At the same time, swing the cane in front of your chest diagonally toward the west with your left palm gently touching the cane to secure it with your right hand. Imagine the cane is an extension of your right forearm. With the tail of the cane, intercept your opponent's weapon and adhere to it. Keep the body of your cane covering your front diagonally, with the cane tail positioned high in front of your head. This posture is derived from the barehand, Yang-style tai chi ward-off posture and forms a solid protection for the upper part of your body (Photo 4-2).

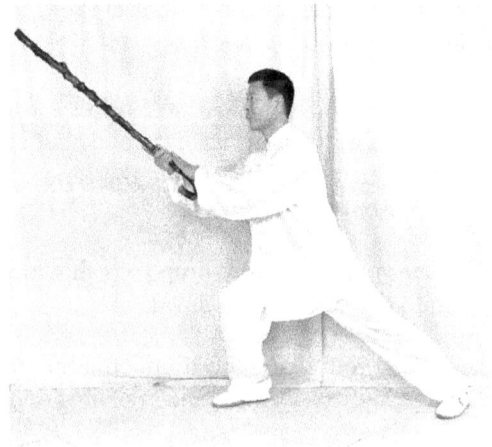

Photo 4-2

Movement 3

Turn your torso slightly toward your left and then shift weight back to your left foot. At the same time, turn the tip of your cane in a counterclockwise circle by flipping your right palm down while your left hand moves to the middle part of the cane to redirect an attack sliding toward your left side. This is a move to defend your center from your right front to left rear in case your opponent is too strong and your ward off in Movement 2 cannot deflect his weapon to your right side. Instead of moving forcefully against him, you will smoothly coil your cane from the left side to the right side of the opponent's weapon to deflect it to the left side of your body. This flipping of the right palm is the same as the barehand form. Turning your torso to the left side is also important to guide the opponent's weapon away from you (Photo 4-3).

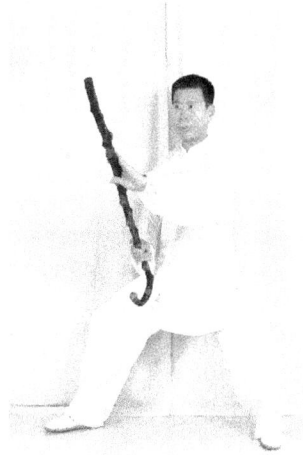

Photo 4-3

Movement 4

Turn your torso to the right again and shift weight forward with the cane horizontally in front of your chest. Press the cane forward with both hands. The horizontal cane serves the same role as your forearms in the barehand form's press. This is the motion to occupy the battlefield and not give the opponent any space to operate his weapon. The best result is to seal your opponent's weapon to his torso (Photo 4-4).

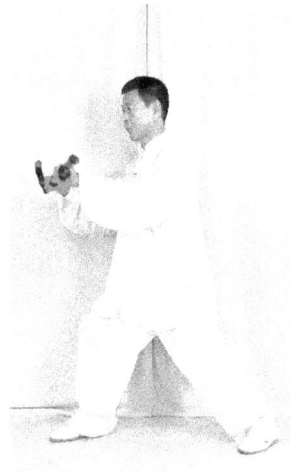

Photo 4-4

Movement 5

Drop the cane a little with a small step behind your right foot into a crouching pose to gather the earth's energy. Sink both hips and keep your center of gravity low (Photo 4-5).

Movement 6

Step your right foot to the right (west) into a large bow stance. Follow up with a big forward strike like a powerful tiger pouncing. The cane is pushed out at your shoulder height. Your arms are fully extended without locking the elbows (Photo 4-6).

Key Points

1) This is a classic Yang-style tai chi posture. Make sure the energy flow is the same as in the barehand form.

2) Pivot at the waist when you turn your body back and forth.

3) Settle your hips down to rebound the earth's energy to power the cane application.

4) Keep a distance of about twelve inches between your heels in the bow stance for good balance and easy energy flow.

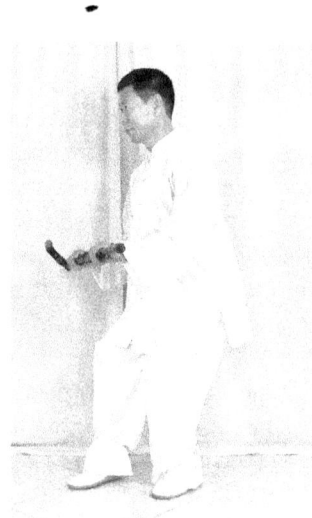

Photo 4-5

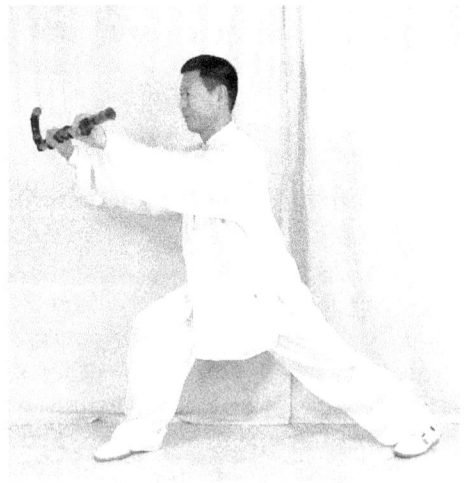

Photo 4-6

Posture 5: Single Whip 單鞭

Movement 1

Following the double-handed pouncing forward move in Grasp Bird's Tail, turn your torso to the left and twist the cane upward toward the left. At the same time, change the cane from a horizontal position to a diagonal position with the cane butt (handle hook) up front. Slide both palms down to the cane tail to use the full extension of the cane in front to target the opponent's neck with the hook (Photo 5-1).

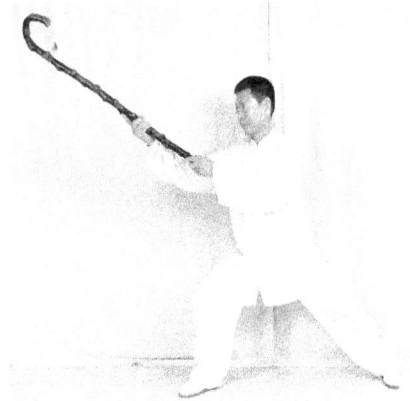

Photo 5-1

Movement 2

As soon as your cane handle hooks the opponent's neck, snap suddenly by shifting your bodyweight back to your left foot. This motion is powered by your torso's movement and not by the movement of your arms (Photo 5-2).

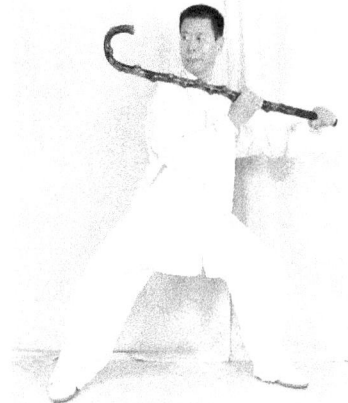

Photo 5-2

Movement 3

Change your grip so that the right knuckles are facing up, and lead the cane with a small counterclockwise circle to clear the space. Shift weight to your right leg, and move your left foot a half step in to create a rebounding momentum to smash the handle end against the opponent's face. The strike is powered by your weight shift toward your right foot (Photo 5-3).

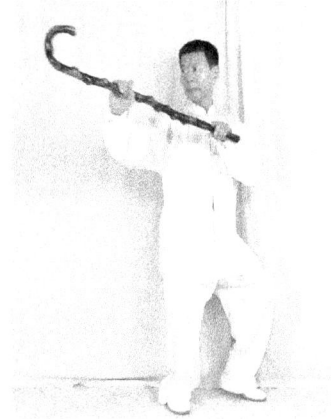

Photo 5-3

Movement 4

Release your left hand from the tail of the cane for an outward parry, holding the cane with only your right hand. With your left hand in front of your chest, look toward your left side (Photo 5-4).

Movement 5

Turn to your left side (east) and roll the cane back to your rear right (southwest). Step out with your left foot, shift weight forward, and bend the left knee into a bow stance. At the same time, push your left hand to the east to finish the Single Whip posture (Photo 5-5).

Key Points

1) Before executing the hooking motion, change the position of your right hand to grab the cane with the palm facing up in order to apply a hook and plucking move. Keep six to eight inches of distance between your palms.

2) Use the handle end to crush the opponent's face. This is a good example of an explosive smashing and crushing application with the cane butt. Make sure the power comes from your torso.

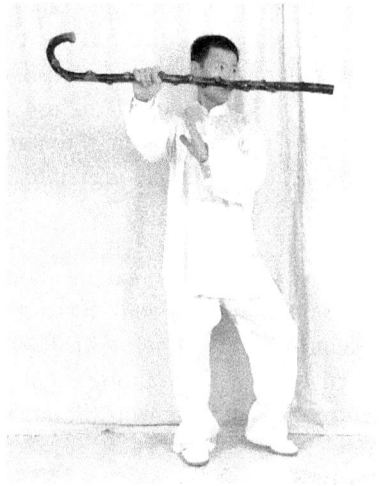

Photo 5-4

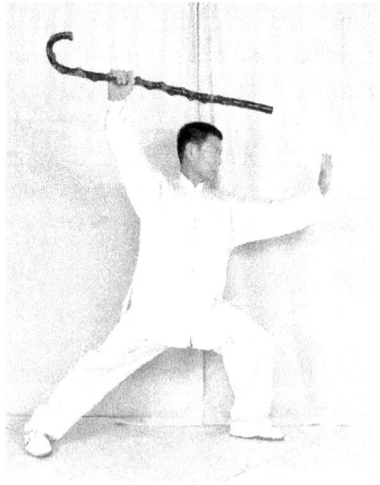

Photo 5-5

Posture 6: Needle Poking Up 海底针

Movement 1
Drop your right hand to the side of your right hip with the cane horizontally guarding your belly. At the same time, shift weight back to your right foot and draw your left forearm back toward your chest (Photo 6-1).

Movement 2
Shift weight forward to your left foot and strike the cane tip down as if to strike your opponent's knee. At the same time, lower your left palm to cover your right elbow area. Finish the pose in a left bow stance (Photo 6-2).

Movement 3
Sink your right hip and shift weight back to the right foot. At the same time, move the cane from lower front to your front centerline and follow the torso turn to shift toward your right while drawing a clockwise curve to roll back the cane. Keep the cane's tail higher above your head as if protecting your front upper area. Your left palm follows your torso turning right to guard your chest (Photo 6-3).

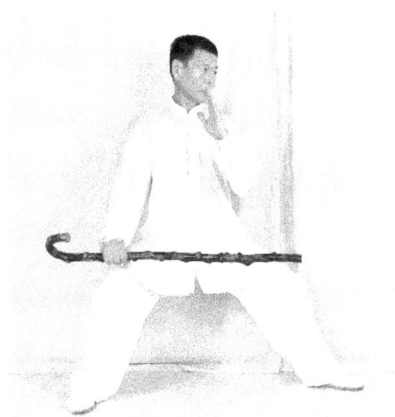

Photo 6-1

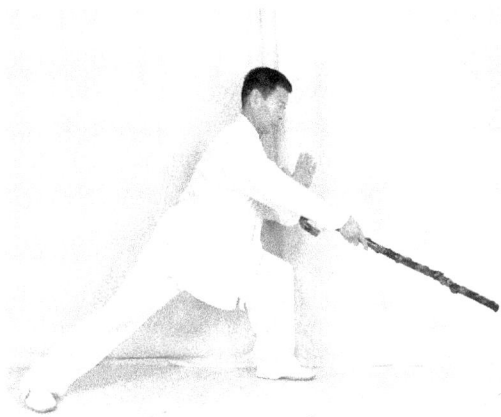

Photo 6-2

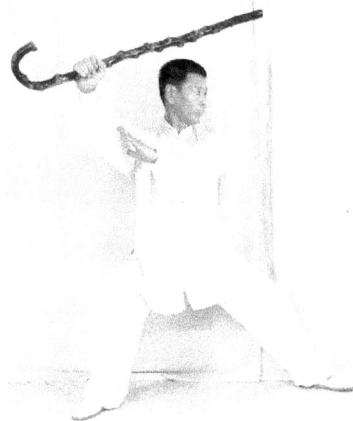

Photo 6-3

Movement 4

Let the cane continue the curve moving toward your right rear with the tail pointing back low. At the same time, shift your weight forward to your left foot, and bend the left knee into a bow stance. Shift your body weight to your left foot and move your left palm in a downward curve and then up in front of your chest to ward off. At the end, the body of the cane is almost parallel with your right leg with your right thumb and index finger extended along the cane (Photo 6-4).

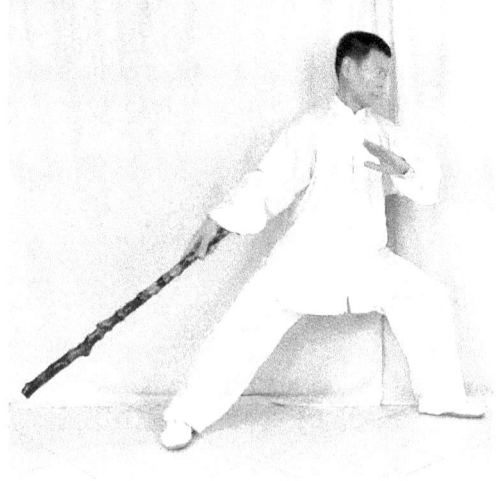

Movement 5

Swing your right hand forward and upward from behind. Move your right foot up a half-step in front. Use your left hand to tap at the cane hook and jerk your right wrist to poke the cane's tail up (Photo 6-5).

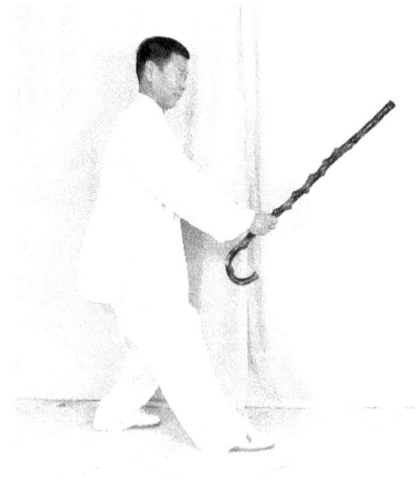

Key Points

1) Use your weight shifting forward to strike the cane low in front, and after the roll back shifting weight to right foot, use the weight flow forward to make the tip of the cane poke up.

2) Sink your buttocks and hips when the cane tilts up. This sinking will rebound the energy from the earth to the cane tip in an upper strike.

Photo 6-4

Photo 6-5

26

Posture 7: White Crane Spreads Wings 白鹤亮翅

Movement 1

Step back with your right foot, drop the tip of the cane to begin a counterclockwise circle in front of your chest. As you twirl the cane, pull the right hand up to use the cane as protection in front of you diagonally with the hook in front of head to the right and the tail in front of your left hip. Your left palm attaches to your right forearm as if to brace your right hand in the cane ward off (Photo-7-1).

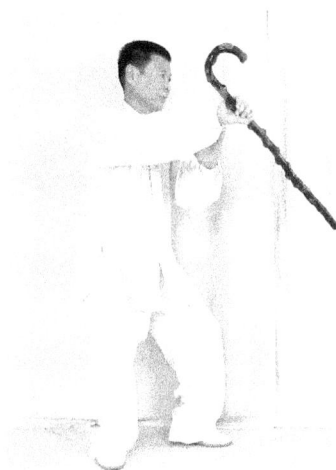

Movement 2

Raise your right hand with your torso slightly turning to the right, as if you are rolling back the cane to redirect an incoming force. At the same time, brush down your left palm and adjust your left foot with toes touching the floor. The cane hook is higher than your head with tip diagonally pointing down in front of your face as if to protect your upper body (Photo 7-2).

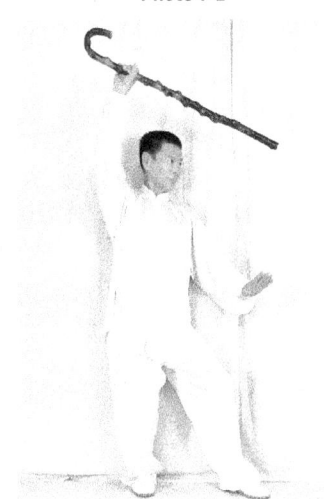

Key Points

1) Use your dantian rotation to twirl the cane in front of your center. It is the belly center that produces the spiral energy that drives your arm and wrist circling.

2) At the finished pose, sink your buttocks and hips while pulling up your spine and head to create an elongated extension of your back.

Photo 7-1

Photo 7-2

Posture 8: Brush Knee 搂膝拗步

Movement 1

Drop your right hand in front of your chest and step your left foot slightly toward the left front. At the same time, put your left palm just above the middle part of the cane to ward off toward your right side while your left foot moves to the left (Photo 8-1).

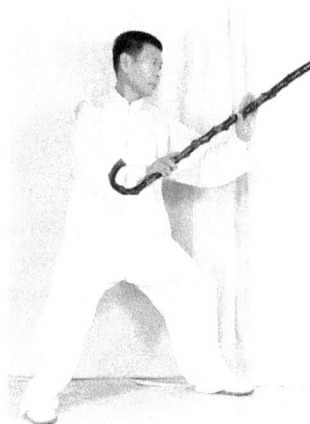

Movement 2

Shift weight forward and pull the left-hand end of the cane back in a clockwise circle from the centerline passing through the front of your left knee. At the same time, tilt up the right-hand end of the cane in front of your right shoulder (Photo 8-2).

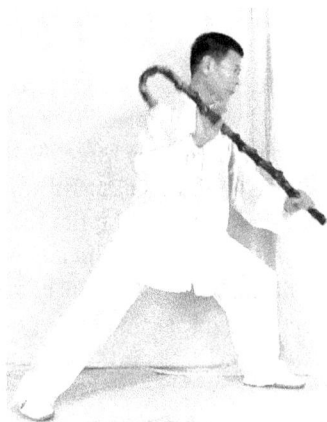

Movement 3

Push your right palm forward to strike the cane hook toward your front centerline. Your left hand holds the tip of the cane back toward the left hip. At the end of the pose, fully extend your right leg and bend your left knee to form a left bow stance (Photo 8-3).

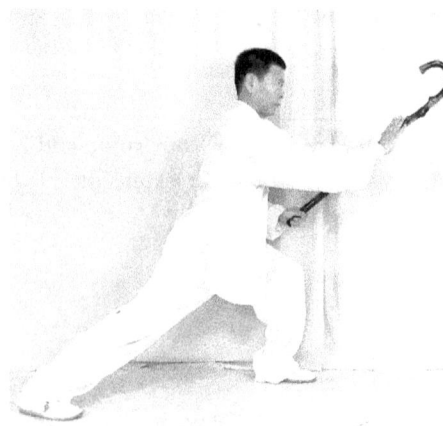

Key Points

1) This is exactly the same as the Brush Knee posture in barehand tai chi. With the cane as the extension of your arm, you can use it to brush off a blade toward your center and strike the hook end to the opponent's chest.

2) Your left hand applies the energy from the extension of your right leg. Therefore, the striking power is a combination of both your hands.

Photo 8-1

Photo 8-2

Photo 8-3

Posture 9: Playing Guitar 手揮琵琶

Movement 1

Move your right foot close to the left heel and shift weight to the right foot. Settle your center of gravity down, and lift the left heel. At the same time, draw the cane hook back with a circular motion to the right side, and push the cane tail forward with your left hand (Photo 9-1).

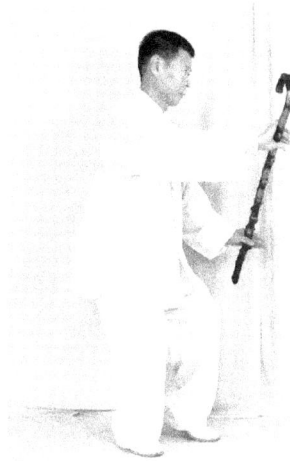

Movement 2

Twist the cane in a clockwise circle in front of your chest. At the same time, pull the cane hook down to the front of your belly, and push the cane tail forward guarding your front centerline. Step your left foot forward a half-step with the heel touching the floor. At the end, the cane is diagonal in front of your body, with the cane tip at face height (Photo 9-2).

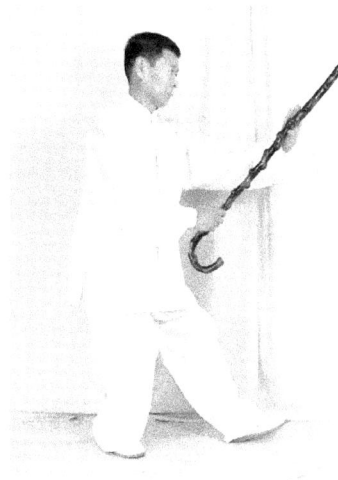

Key Points

1) The twisting power is from your torso, not from your arms.

2) End with a left empty stance. Your left heel rests on the floor lightly with the potential ability to kick up.

Photo 9-1

Photo 9-2

Posture 10: Diagonal Flying 斜飛势

Movement 1

Move the cane tail in an arc from your front center down towards your right front, while stepping with your left foot towards the left front corner. The cane ends low at the right side of your hips (Photo 10-1).

Movement 2

Swing the cane tail to your right and strike up in a counterclockwise arc from the lower right to your upper left front while shifting weight forward to your left foot. Bend your left knee into a left bow stance. The cane is diagonally across your left front with the cane handle guarding the chest and the tail higher in front of your head. The cane is parallel to your right leg. Turn your head to face the right (Photo 10-2).

Key Points

1) The cane is moved in an oval shape diagonally in front of you. Make sure to move the cane down to the right then up to the left.

2) The power to swing the cane to the left front is driven by your right foot and torso's motion.

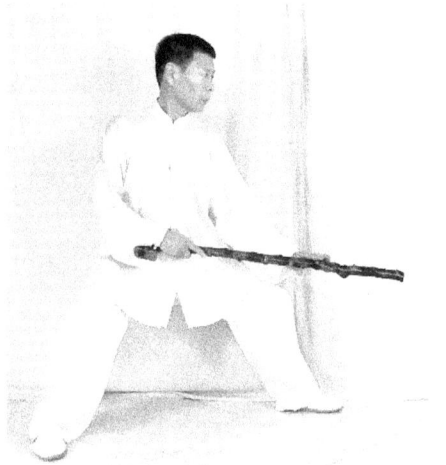

Photo 10-1

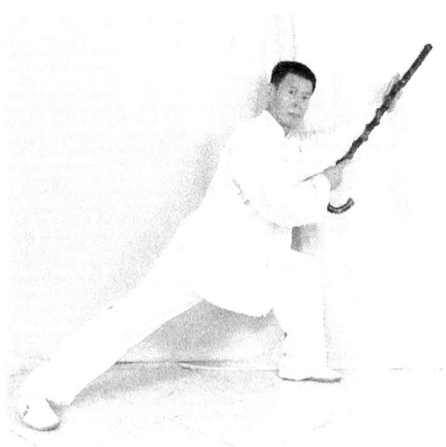

Photo 10-2

Posture 11: Deflect, Parry, and Jab Cane 搬攔杖

Movement 1

Turn your torso to the left side by pivoting on your left heel while turning the cane counterclockwise from the right side to your left side. Draw your right foot from behind up in front of your left foot a few inches to store up energy with both knees bending slightly. Draw the cane in front of your chest and sink your hips as if you were a crouching tiger (Photo 11-1).

Movement 2

Step your right foot forward and jab the cane hook straight forward. The cane is diagonal with the hook end higher. Slide the left hand to the tail of the cane in front of your chest (Photo 11-2, 11-2, front and back).

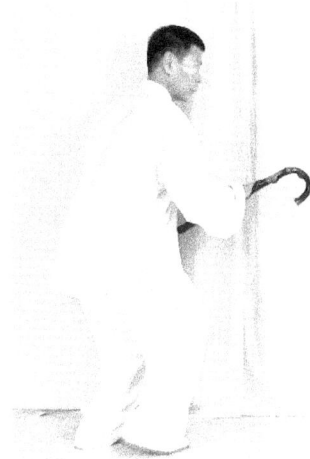

Photo 11-1

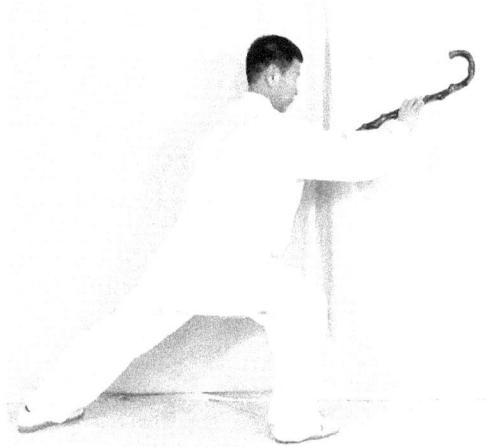

Photo 11-2

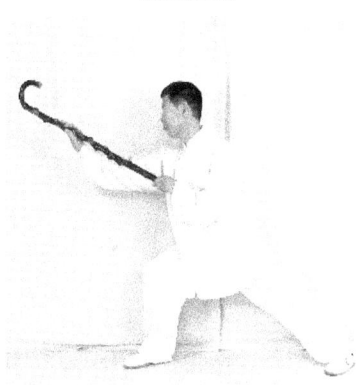

(Photo 11-2 Back View)

Movement 3

Shift your weight back to your left foot and withdraw your right foot halfway back, while pulling the cane back toward your left side with your palms sliding to the hook end to spin the tail from your left side to your front center. The tail is at face height guarding your front (Photo 11-3).

Movement 4

Without a stop, deflect the cane tail from your center toward your lower right side while stepping your right foot behind your left. The cane follows your right foot pulling back and guards the outside of your right leg. Your chest turns to your right in the southeast direction as you step your right foot back, but your eyes are still looking to the east (Photo 11-4). (Note: Movements 3 and 4 can be played in a continuous manner without a pause in between.)

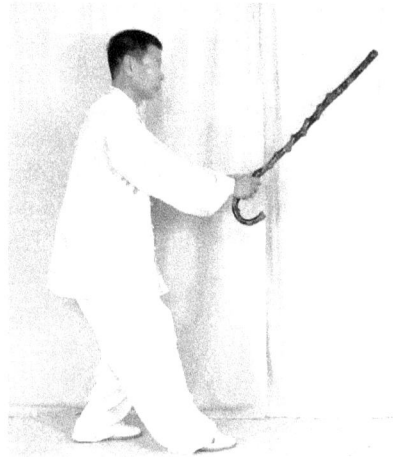
Photo 11-3

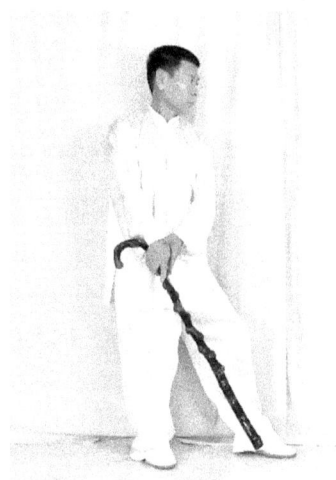
Photo 11-4

Movement 5

Swing the cane from your lower right side across your center front high and then to your lower left side to protect the side of your left leg. Use your torso's turn to drive the cane's swing (Photo 11-5).

Movement 6

Spin the tail of the cane from your left side low up in front of your body, and then twist your right hand at the wrist to twirl the cane in a circle at your right side. At the same time, lift your right foot up. Use your torso's twisting motion from left and right to power the cane circling at your left and right (Photo 11-6).

Movement 7

As soon as you finish the cane twist circle on your right side, land your right foot in front with the toes pointing to the southeast, so your chest faces to the southeast (Photo 11-7).

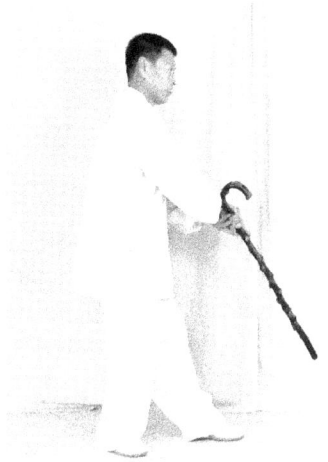

Photo 11-5

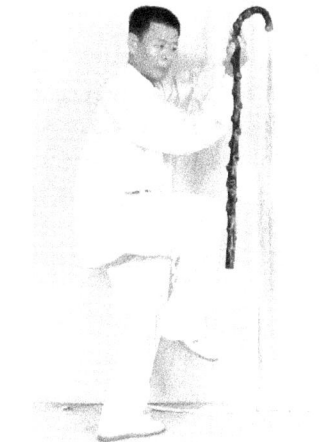

Photo 11-6

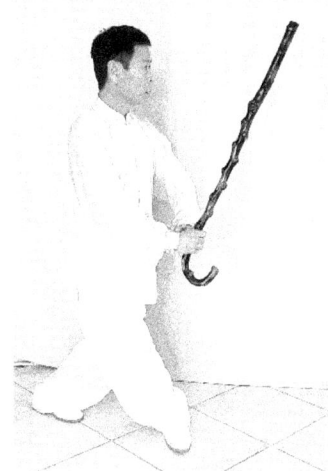

Photo 11-7

Movement 7

Step your left foot forward with the cane guarding in front of you with the handle hook at your belly level and the tail pointing forward at chin height. Your left palm is protected in front of your chest. You can also use a jumping step here to leap your right foot forward and immediately land the left foot in front. Keep your weight on the right foot at the end of this move (Photo 11-7).

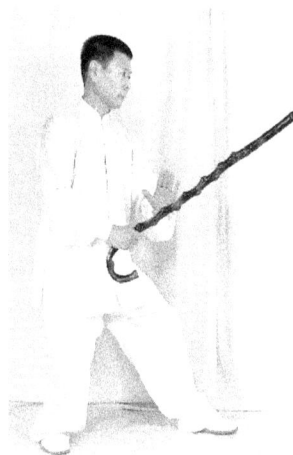

Movement 8

Shift weight forward to your left foot and bend the left knee into a left bow stance. At the same time, strike the cane tail directly forward. The cane is lined up with your right arm at shoulder height. Your left hand and the cane handle move forward together (Photo 11-8).

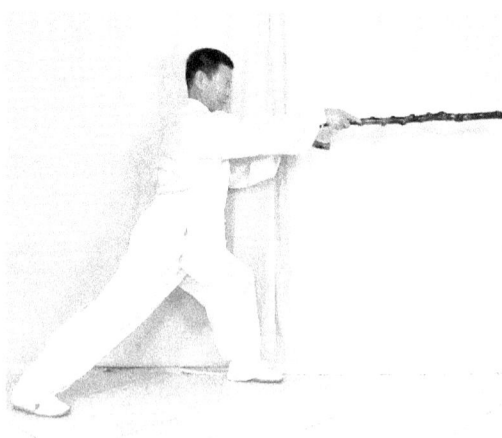

Photo 11-7

Key Points

1) The first jab employs the cane hook toward the opponent's chin as if an uppercut strike. The second strike employs the cane tail toward his heart. In between these two strikes, swing the cane across your front center twice to deflect the incoming attacks.

2) The optional jumping step can be used to cover a long distance to reach your opponent, or to jump up high enough to avoid his attack toward your knee. While you are leaping in the air, twirl the cane to protect your leg.

Photo 11-8

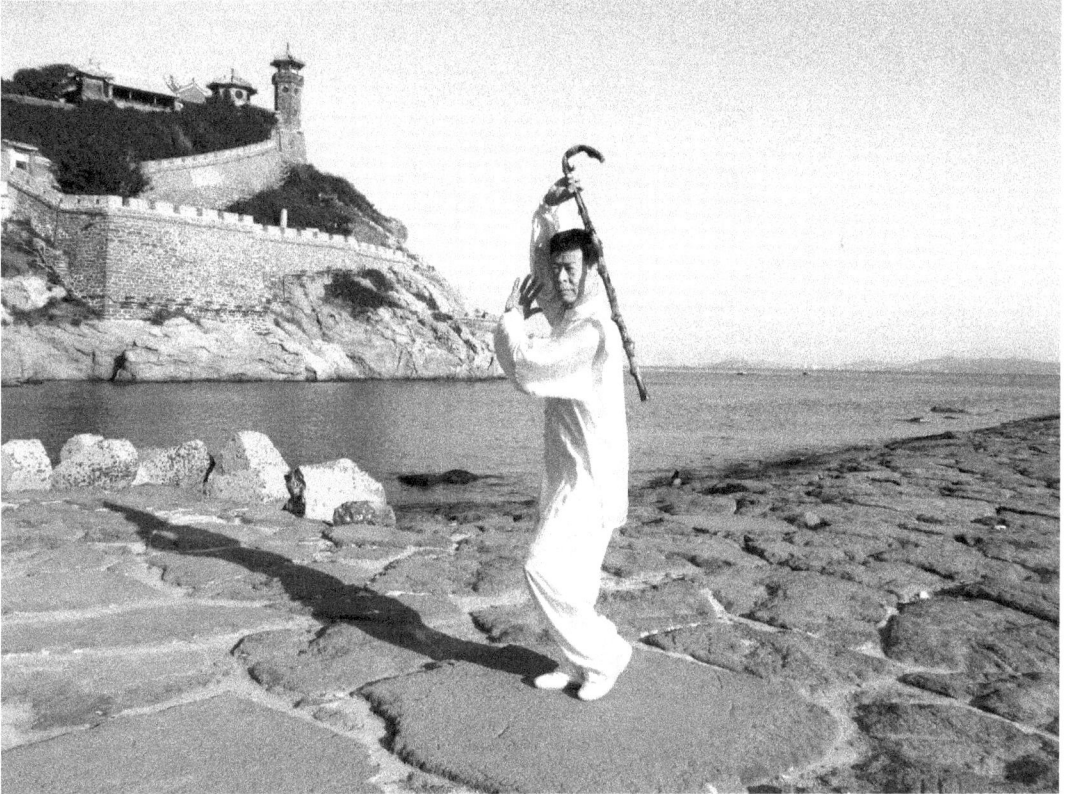

纏頭杖

Wrap Cane
Around Head

Posture 12: Dragon Swirling Tail 乌龍攬尾

Movement 1

Drop the cane tail and turn the cane from the right side in a counterclockwise circle while withdrawing your weight back to your right foot and pulling back your left foot a half step with the left heel up and toes touching the floor. Your torso twist leads the cane swirl. Body and cane are united together in this move. At the end of this posture, the handle of the cane is higher above your head than the cane tail, which protects at face level (Photo 12-1).

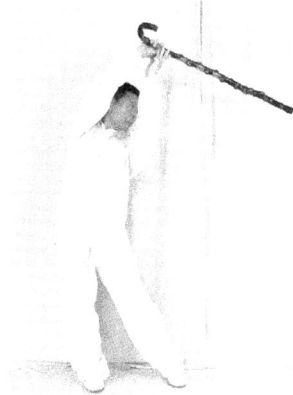

Photo 12-1

Movement 2

Step your left foot back and shift your weight onto it. Lift the right heel with right toes lightly touching the floor. Turn and twist your torso to your left side to lead the cane in a clockwise circle to deflect any incoming attacks to your left (Photo 12-2).

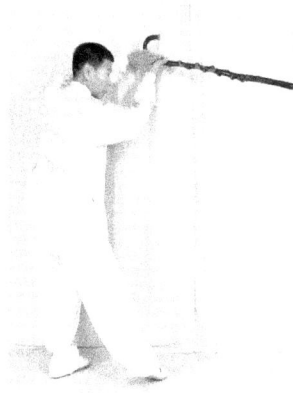

Movement 3

Step your right foot back and shift your weight onto your right foot. Lift the left heel with left toes lightly touching the floor. Turn and twist your torso to your right side to lead the cane in a counterclockwise circle to deflect any incoming attacks to your right side. This movement is the reverse of the previous Movement 12-2 (Photo 12-3).

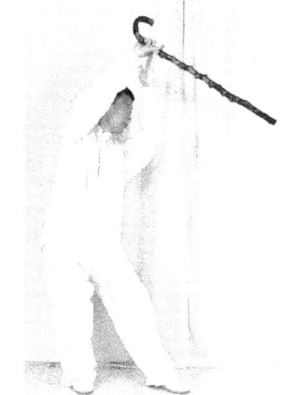

Photo 12-2

Key Points

1) This protective retreat technique allows you to stay away from an aggressive attacker. Twirl the cane in front of you while you are stepping back.

2) You can take more backward steps if you have the space in your practice area. The cane is like a dragon's swirling tail. Your coiling torso initiates the motion of your arms and the cane is the extension of your arm.

Photo 12-3

Posture 13: Needle Hiding in Curling Lotus Leaf 葉底藏针

Movement 1

Adjust your left foot with the toes curved inward, or twist your left heel outward by pivoting on your left toes and turn your torso backward while keeping the cane above your head pointing to the front. Your head is under the cover of the cane with your eyes looking at the cane tail (Photo 13-1).

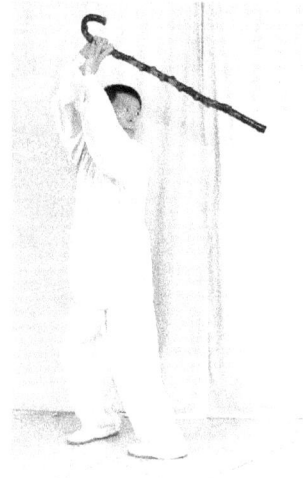

Photo 13-1

Movement 2

Continue to twist your left foot by pivoting on the heel, and turn your torso to your right. Step your right foot in a back curve to the northeast corner with right toes lightly resting on the floor. Drop your hands to chin level and hold the cane horizontally in front of you with the tail of the cane still pointing to the right front (Photo 13-2).

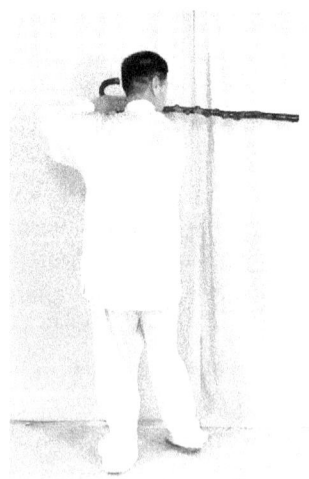

Photo 13-2

Movement 3

Step your right foot toward the east and hold the cane at shoulder height aiming to your right side with your right palm facing your right shoulder. At the same time, ward off with your left palm to the west side to balance the cane pointing to the east side (Photo 13-3).

Movement 4

Lift your left leg and foot to protect your crotch. Push your left palm to the cane hook to strike the tip of the cane to the east side at shoulder height. At the same time, turn your right hand counterclockwise to create a drilling motion at the tip of the cane, ending with your right palm facing downward and your right arm totally extended (Photo 13-4 and 13-4b, reversed pose).

Key Points

1) When you turn your torso from front facing to back facing, keep the cane constantly on top of your head and keep the tip pointing to your opponent.

2) When you strike with the tip of the cane, make sure to fully extend your right arm to create a firm structure to launch the thrust.

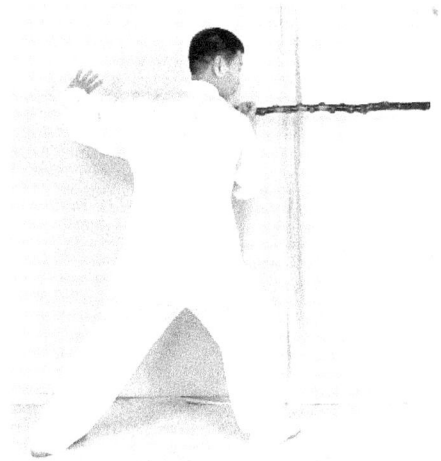

Photo 13-3

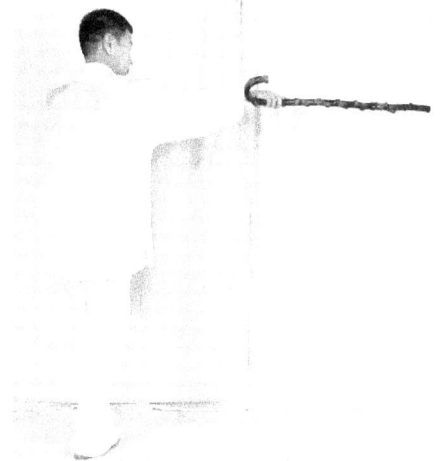

Photo 13-4

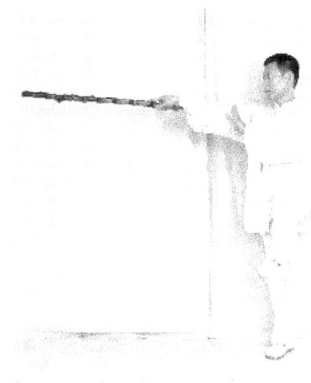

Photo 13-4b (reversed pose)

Posture 14: Wrap Cane Around Head 纏頭杖

Posture 1

Step your left foot down to the west side and shift weight to your left foot. Bend your left knee into a bow stance and turn your head to face the west. At the same time, ward off your left forearm in front of your chest and drop the cane behind (the east side). Keep the cane in a diagonal line with your right arm (Photo 14-1 and 14-1b back and front view).

Posture 2

Step to the northwest corner with your right foot, toes pointing a little outward. At the same time, swing the cane alongside as the right foot steps as if to protect the right leg. Continue to move the cane from the lower front right (northwest) across your torso to the upper left outside your left shoulder (southwest) with the handle higher than your head and the tip at chest level pointing down (Photo 14-2).

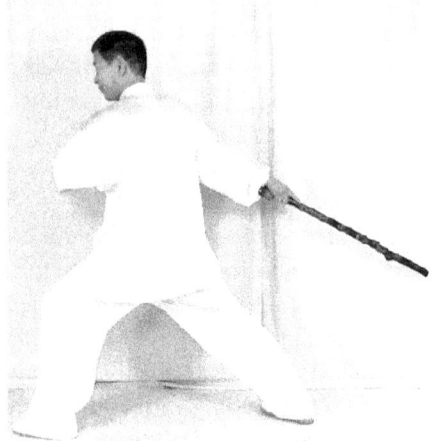

Photo 14-1

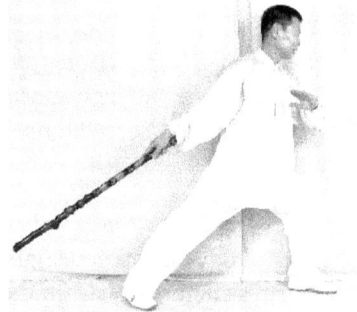

Photo 14-1b (front view)

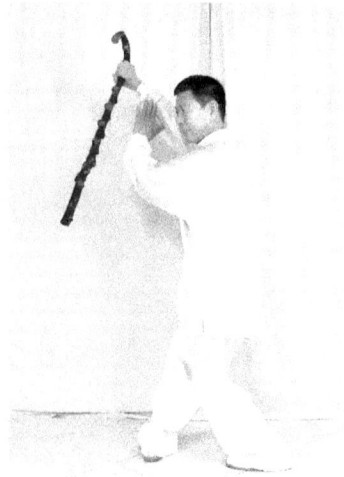

Photo 14-2

Movement 3

Continue to wrap the cane from outside your left shoulder across the back of your head to the back of your right shoulder. At the same time, step your left foot to the southwest direction and bend the left knee. The cane on your right shoulder protects the right side of your head, and your left forearm is warding off in front of your chest (Photo 14-3).

Movement 4

Strike the cane down in front of you while lifting your left palm in front of your forehead to balance the cane's downward striking motion. Face to the west, but the cane strikes slightly toward the northwest corner direction (Photo 14-4).

Key Points

1) Turn the cane around your head in a complete circle from the lower right back to the upper right side before chopping down. The wrapping motion is powered by your torso twist.

2) For energy balance, coordinate striking down the cane and lifting the left palm.

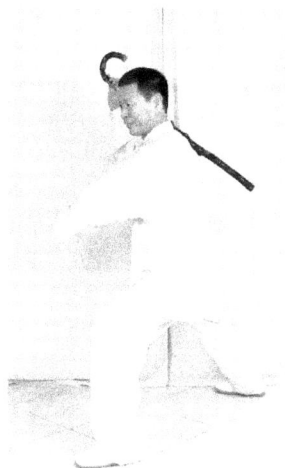

Photo 14-3

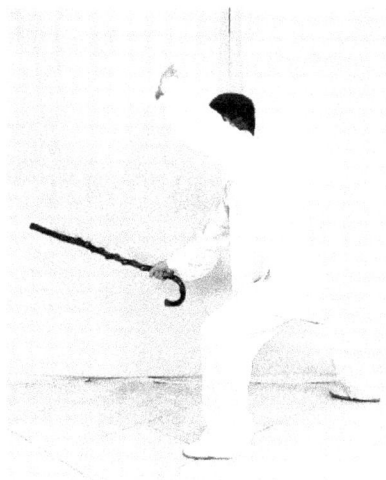

Photo 14-4

Posture 15: Fair Lady Works Shuttle in Four Corner Directions 玉女穿梭

Movement 1

Turn your torso to your left to lead the cane sweeping across your front centerline as if to redirect an incoming weapon from your left side with the cane guarding the outside of your left arm. At the same time, pull your right foot toward the left foot and shift weight to your right foot with the ball of your left foot lightly touching the floor. Keep both hips unlocked, bending knees slightly. This movement is a left empty stance facing the southwest corner (Photo 15-1).

Movement 2

Keep the cane guarding outside your left arm as a shield. Step your left foot and bump your left shoulder to power the cane in a ramming motion to the southwest corner. Finish this move with a left bow stance (Photo 15-2).

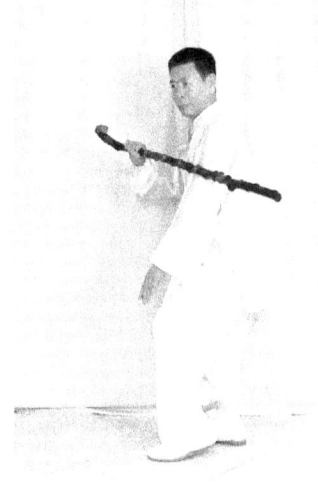

Photo 15-1

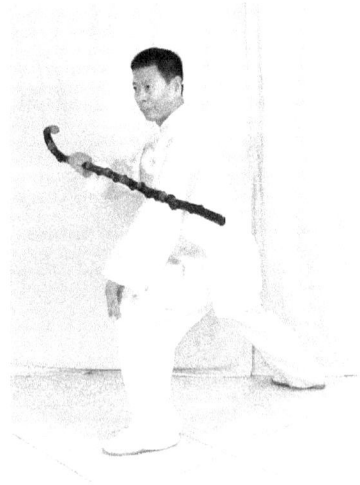

Photo 15-2

Movement 3

Toss the lower part of the cane off your left arm and catch it with your left hand about five to six inches above the tip end. Keep the cane diagonally in front of your chest with your right hand holding the hook end at your head height and the cane tip at waist height. Transfer your left bow stance into a horseback riding stance with the cane warding off to the southwest corner (Photo 15-3).

Movement 4

Turn your torso toward your right and turn your left foot inward to facilitate your torso's turning. Shift body weight to your right foot and bend your right knee with the left leg stretched. At the same time, smash the cane hook toward the northeast corner at face height. Loosely hold the cane in your right hand, releasing your fingers and sliding down a little from the cane handle end with the cane held in the valley between the thumb and index finger. Grab the cane firmly with your left hand in front of your chest. Turn your torso 180 degrees from the southwest to northeast (Photo 15-4).

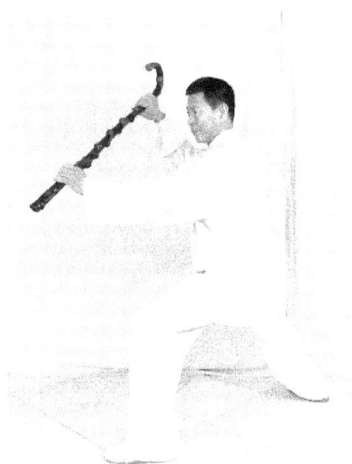

Photo 15-3

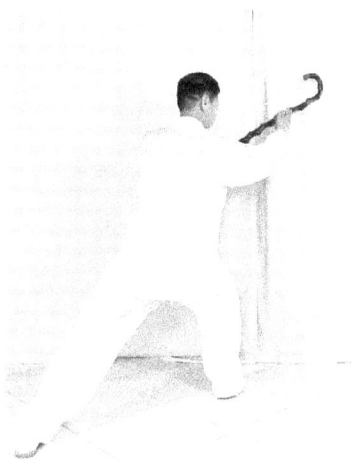

Photo 15-4

Movement 5

Shift weight to your left foot and pull your right foot back with toes touching the floor into a right empty stance. At the same time, draw your right hand back and lower the cane handle as if to deflect/redirect an incoming weapon away from your torso (Photo 15-5).

Movement 6

Pivot on the ball of your right foot and turn your torso to your right with your left heel sliding back to facilitate your body's turn. At the same time, spin the cane clockwise with the left hand end up from your left side (Photo 15-6). Without stopping, step toward the southeast corner with your right foot and bend your right knee into a bow stance. Strike the cane tail at face height with your left palm pressing on the top of the cane and your right hand holding the cane near the hook in front of the right hip (Photo 15-7).

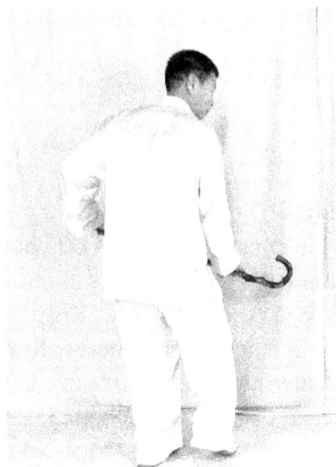

Photo 15-5

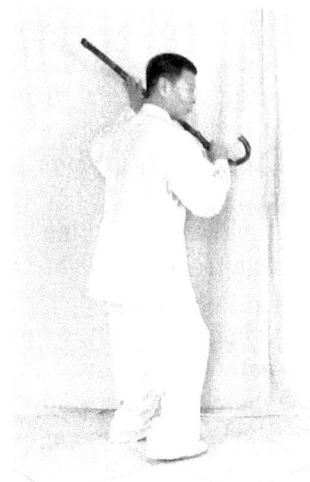

Photo 15-6

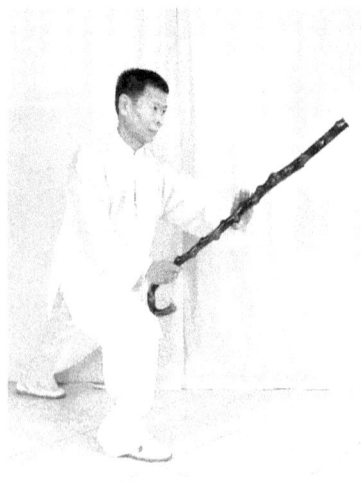

Photo 15-7

Movement 7

This movement is almost the same as Movement 1. Turn your torso to your left to lead the cane sweeping across your front centerline as if to redirect an incoming weapon to the left with the cane guarding outside your left arm. At the same time, pull your left foot toward the right foot with the ball of your left foot lightly touching the floor. Keep both hips unlocked, bending knees slightly. This is a left empty stance facing the northeast corner (Photo 15-8).

Movement 8

This movement is the same as Movement 2, except you strike in the opposite direction. Keep the cane as a shield guarding outside your left arm, step out with your left foot, and bump your left shoulder to power the cane ramming hit to the northeast corner. Finish this move with a left bow stance (Photo 15-9).

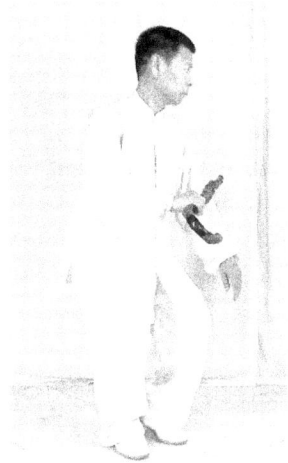

Photo 15-8

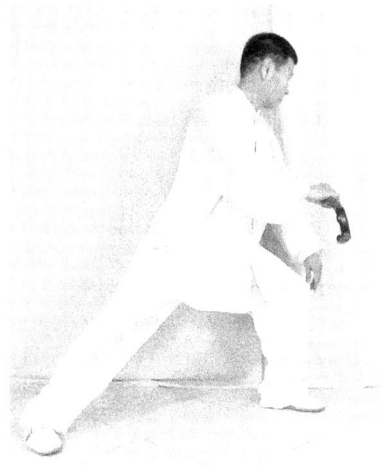

Photo 15-9

Movement 9

This movement is the same as Movement 3, except you strike in the opposite direction. Toss the lower part of the cane off your left arm and catch it with your left hand about five to six inches above the tip end. Keep the cane diagonally in front of your chest with the hook end at head height and the tip at waist level. Transfer your bow stance into a horseback riding stance with the cane warding off to the northeast corner (Photo 15-10).

Movement 10

This movement is the same as Movement 4, except you strike in the opposite direction. Turn your torso toward your right and turn your left foot with the toes curved inward to facilitate your torso's turning. Shift body weight to your right foot, and bend your right knee with the left leg stretched. At the same time, smash the cane hook toward the southwest corner at face height. Hold the cane loosely with your right hand, releasing fingers and sliding down a little from the cane handle end, with the cane held at the valley between the thumb and index finger. Grab the cane firmly with your left hand in front of your chest. Turn your torso 180 degrees from the northeast to southwest (Photo 15-11).

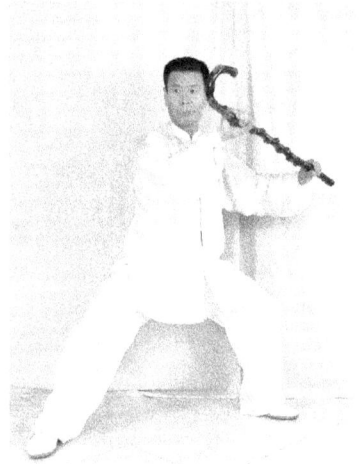

Photo 15-10

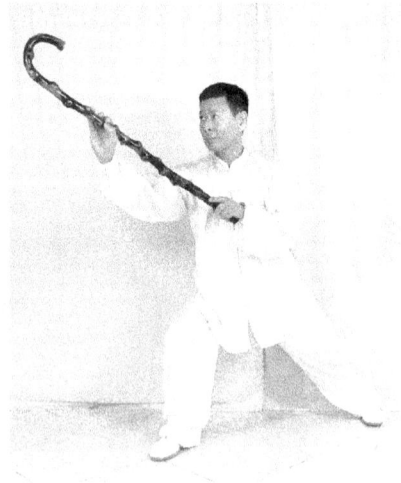

Photo 15-11

Movement 11

This movement is the same as Movement 5, except you strike in the opposite direction. Shift weight to your left foot and pull your right foot back with toes touching the floor in a right empty stance. At the same time, draw your right hand back and lower the cane handle as if to deflect/redirect an incoming weapon from your torso (Photo 15-12).

Movement 12

This movement is the same as Movement 6, except you strike in the opposite direction. Pivot on the ball of your right foot and turn your torso to your right with your left heel sliding back to facilitate your body's right turn. At the same time, spin the cane clockwise with the left-hand end up from your left side. Without stopping, step toward the northeast corner with your right foot and bend your right knee into a right bow stance, striking the cane tail at face height with your left palm pressing on the top of the cane and your right hand holding the cane near the hook in front of the right hip (Photo 15-13).

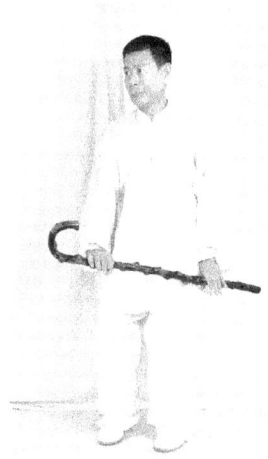

Photo 15-12

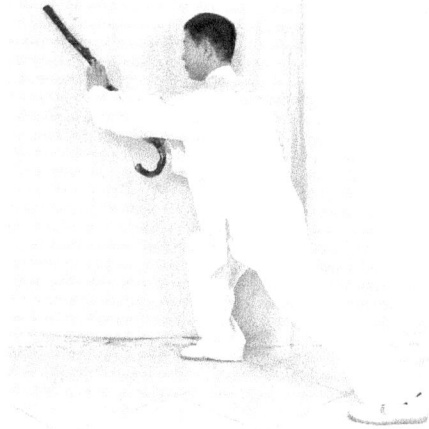

Photo 15-13

Movement 13

This movement is almost the same as Movement 1. Turn your torso to your left to lead the cane sweeping across your front centerline as if to redirect an incoming weapon left with the cane guarding outside your left arm. At the same time, pull your left foot toward your right foot with the left front ball lightly touching the floor. Keep both hips unlocked, bending knees slightly. This is a left empty stance facing the southwest corner (Photo 15-14).

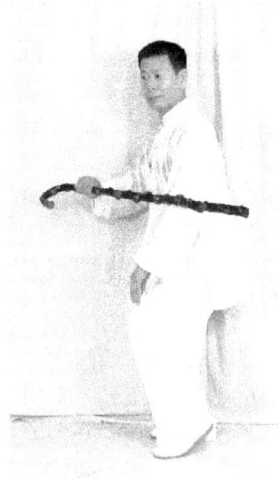

Movement 14

This movement is exactly the same as Movement 2. Keep the cane guarding outside your left arm as a shield, step out with your left foot, and bump your left shoulder to power the cane ramming hit to the southwest corner. Finish this move with your left knee bent and your right leg stretched into a bow stance (Photo 15-15).

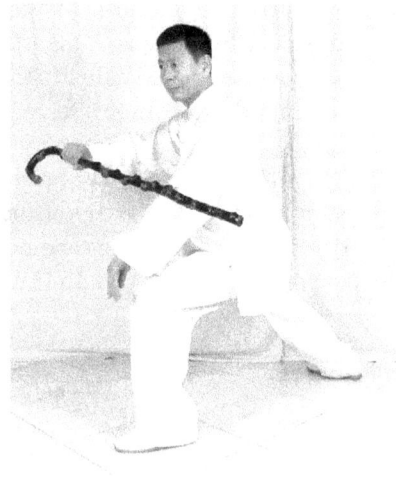

Photo 15-14

Key Points

1) This posture has many repetitive movements. It covers all four corners with shove, jab, and smash, starting and ending from the southwest corner.

2) During the movements, use your feet as the pivot point to facilitate your torso's turning.

3) Make sure the front hand slides along the cane to let the strikes reach the targets.

Photo 15-15

Posture 16: Circle Sweep and High Pat on Horse 高探馬

Movement 1

Turn your left toes inward by pivoting on the left heel to drive your torso to your right. Straighten your body from the left bow stance and draw your right foot close to the left foot. At the same time, raise the cane to your shoulder height to guard your front with the tip point at the southwest corner. Your left hand moves up with the palm near the right wrist area (Photo 16-1).

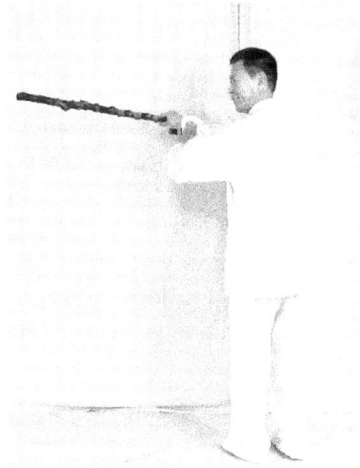

Movement 2

Turn your left heel outward by pivoting on the left ball and turn your torso to your right. At the same time, sweep and hit the cane in a horizontal circle to your right. Keep the left palm around the right wrist as if to support your right hand for the circling strike. Keep the cane at least shoulder height because you are targeting the opponent's neck or head (Photo 16-2).

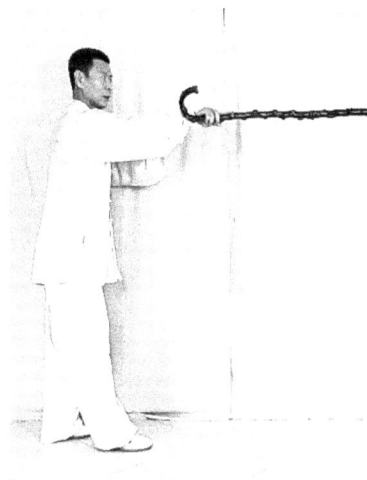

Photo 16-1

Photo 16-2

Movement 3

As you sweep the cane in a circle, draw your right foot to the side of your left foot. Wrap the cane around your head with another small circle with the handle above your head and the cane tip pointing down. This small circle is from your right rear corner across the back of your head and wraps outside your left shoulder, then across the front of your torso and lands the cane tip on the floor a few inches from your right toes. Next, move your left foot a half step forward with the front ball touching the floor. At the same time, push your left palm forward at shoulder height and look forward through your fingertips. You are facing east (Photo 16-3 and 16-4).

Key Points

1) Pull in your right foot to keep your torso vertical when you make the circle-sweep hit. Keep your right arm extended to line up with the cane to make as large a circle as you can to clear the area around you. Imagine swinging the cane to keep a group of opponents away from you.

2) The small circle is different. Keep the cane in a vertical position to wrap around your head and torso for protection.

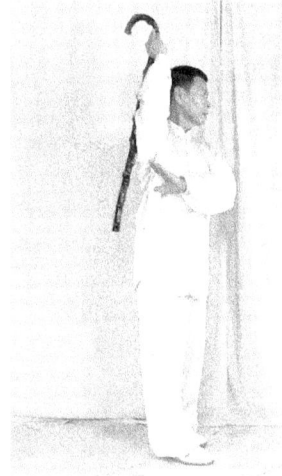

Photo 16-3

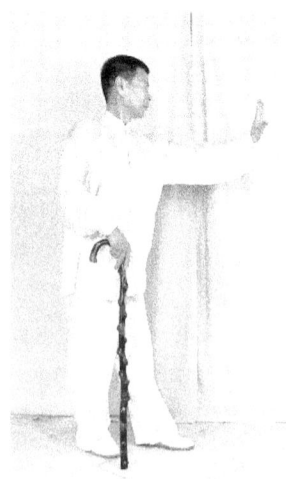

Photo 16-4

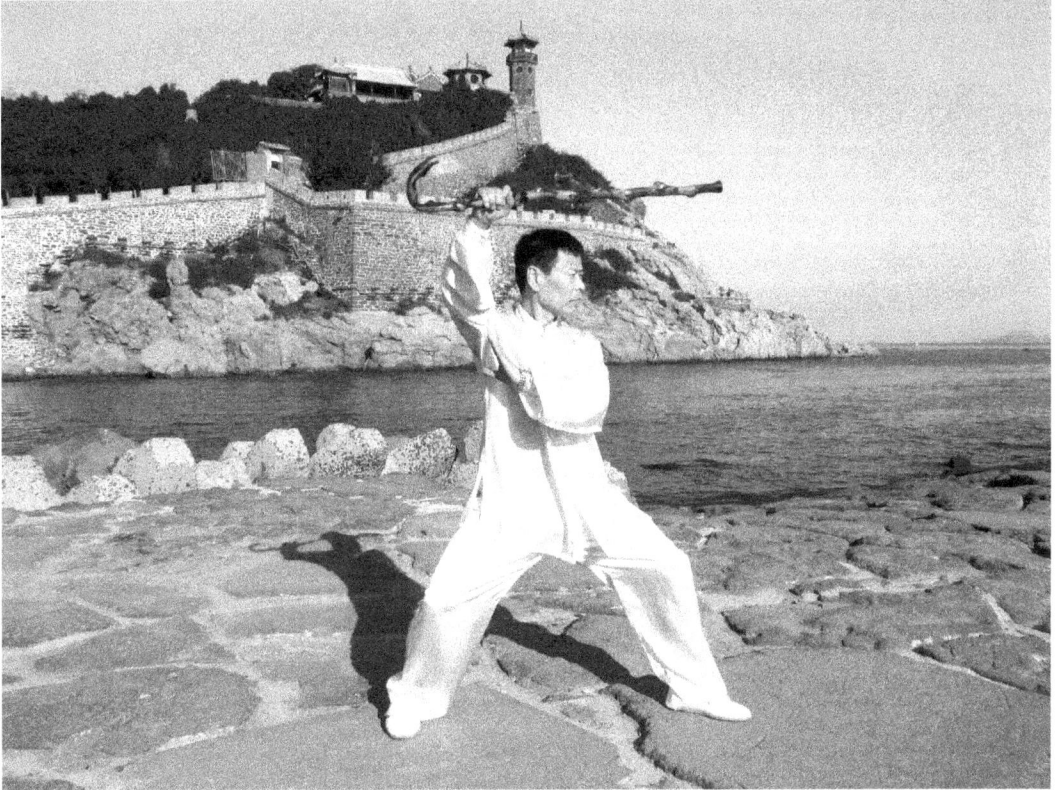

雲手

Cloud Hands

Section III

Posture 17: Wild Horse Kicks Out Hoof 野馬撩蹄

Movement 1

Step your left foot back behind your right heel and squat down. At the same time, parry your left palm toward the right chest and then press the left palm down (Photo 17-1). Optionally, you can squat totally down with the left knee touching the floor and your buttocks sitting on your left heel. This movement is called the *xie-bu*, the resting stance in tai chi practice (Photo 17-1b optional).

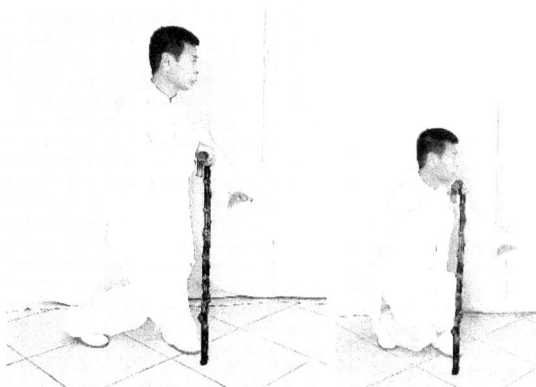

Photo 17-1

Photo 17-1b (optional)

Movement 2

Get up from the lower position and use your right foot to kick the cane tail off the floor so the cane tip strikes upward and forward. At the same time, jerk your right wrist to force the cane handle downward to facilitate the cane tip strike (Photo 17-2).

Optional, Hold the cane with your left hand in front of the right hand, and use the left hand as a fulcrum to pivot the cane tip up (Photo 17-2b optional).

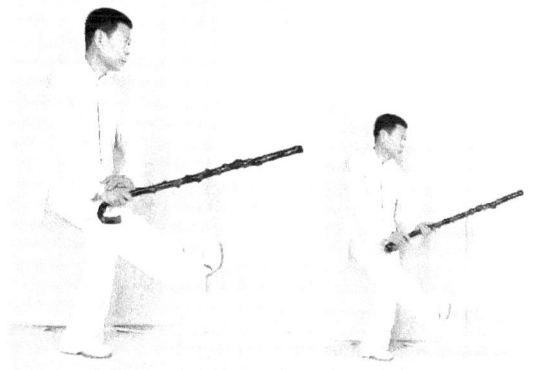

Photo 17-2

Photo 17-2b (optional)

Key Points

1) To form the resting stance, make sure your right toes open toward the southeast corner to open the right hip which allows the left hip to close in. This adjustment will enable the left knee to go across under your right knee.

2) Keep the right foot in that angled position when you make the kick.

Posture 18: Blue Dragon Out of Water 青龍出水

Movement 1

Land your right foot after the kick while twirling the cane tip in a clockwise circle in front of your torso for protection. Immediately step forward with your left foot. Keep the cane guarding at chest height with the tip pointing forward to the east (Photo 18-1).

Movement 2

Shift weight forward to your left foot, bend your left knee, and stretch the right leg into a bow stance. At the same time, thrust the cane tip straight forward to the east with both arms extended. The cane is lined up with your right arm at shoulder height (Photo 18-2).

Key Points

1) Circle the cane in front of you like a dragon twirling to train your inner energy coiling strength. Use your left hand as a fulcrum to pivot the cane tail's circle.

2) Press your right foot to the floor to initiate the forward thrust, and use your torso's movement to power the strike.

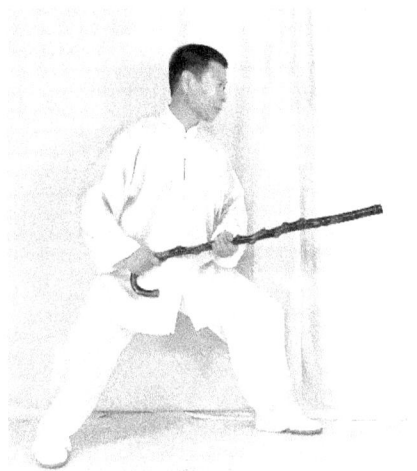

Photo 18-1

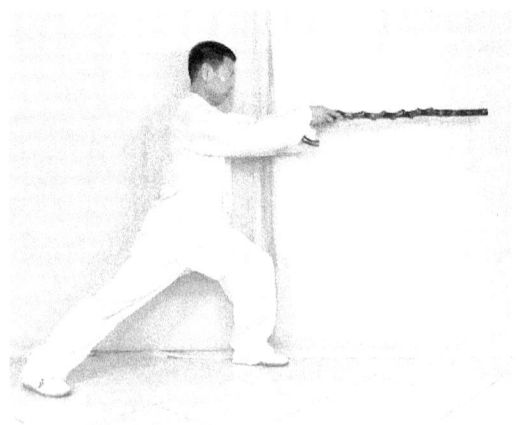

Photo 18-2

Posture 19: Part Wild Horse's Mane 野馬分鬃

Movement 1

Shift weight back to your right foot, parry the cane upward, and draw a rainbow curve back to the front of your right shoulder. At the same time, move your right hand to the middle of the cane and keep the left hand in the handle area. Look to the east (Photo 19-1).

Movement 2

Circle the cane backward and downward to the outside of your right leg with the right hand lower as if you are protecting your right side. At the same time, pull the right leg up and step forward to the east while swinging the cane tip forward and upward. The cane tip reaches out at the level of your head (Photo 19-2).

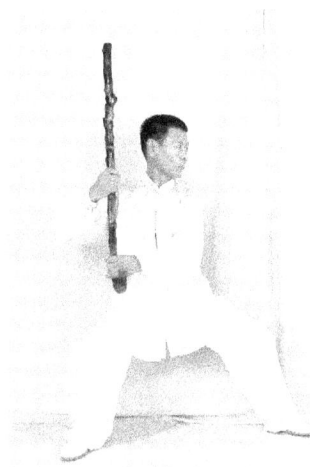

Photo 19-1

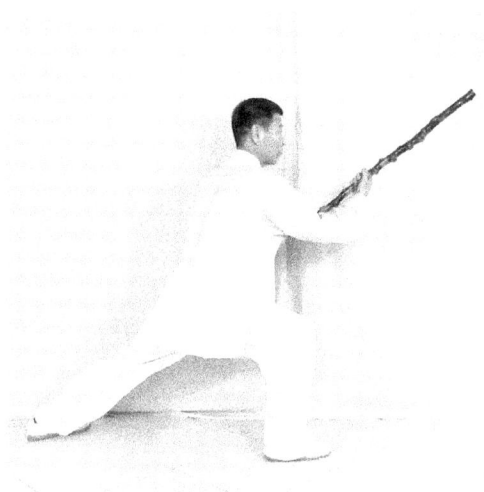

Photo 19-2

Movement 3

Shift weight back to your left foot and parry the cane in a rainbow curve back to the front of your left shoulder. At the same time, switch your left hand up, hold the middle part of the cane, and move your right hand down to the handle area. Look to the east (Photo 19-3).

Movement 4

Circle the cane backward and downward to the outside of your left leg with the left hand lower as if you are protecting your left side (Photo 19-4). Next, step forward to the east with your left foot as you swing the cane tip forward and upward. The cane tip reaches out to the level of your head (Photo 19-5).

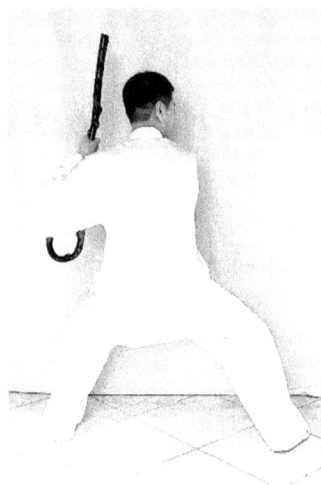

Photo 19-3

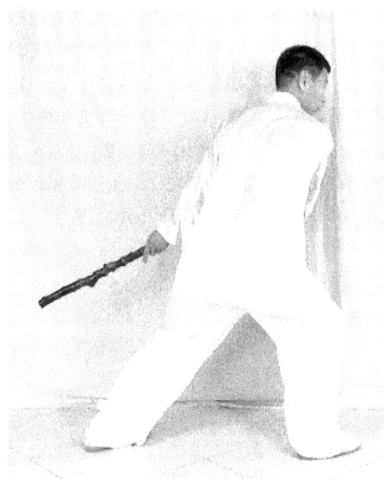

Photo 19-4

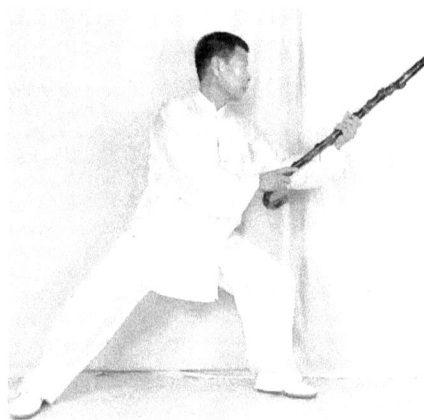

Photo 19-5

Movement 5

Repeat Movement 1. Shift weight back to your right foot and parry the cane in a rainbow curve back to the front of your right shoulder while moving your right hand to the middle part of the cane and sliding the left hand to the handle area. Look to the east (Photo 19-6).

Movement 6

Repeat Movement 2. Circle the cane backward and downward to the outside of your right leg with the right hand lower as if you are protecting your right side. At the same time, step forward to the east with your right foot as you swing the cane tip forward and upward. The cane tip reaches out at the level of your head (Photo 19-7).

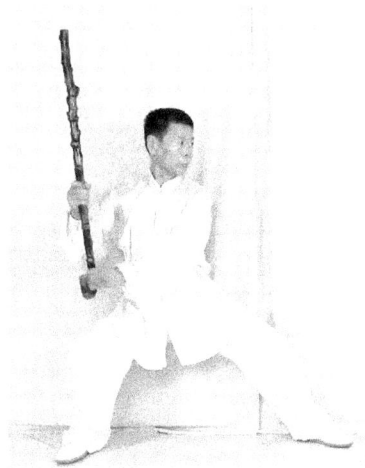

Photo 19-6

Key Points

1) The three steps forward to the east linked with the cane swinging in vertical circles protects you from side to side. The primary purpose is to use the cane as a tool to protect your stepping, and the secondary function is the uppercut swing strike.

2) Switch the position of your hands on the cane position in each step to ensure the cane swings forward smoothly.

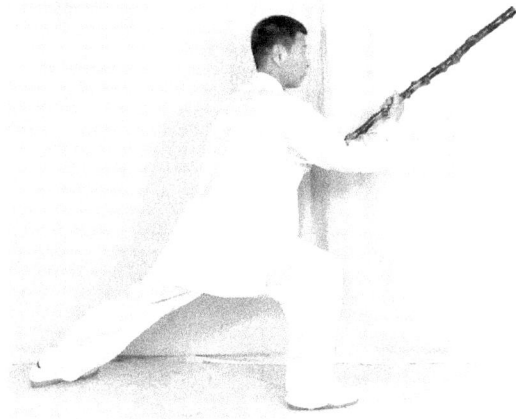

Photo 19-7

Posture 20: Apparent Close 如封似闭

Movement 1

Shift weight back to your left foot and lift the right knee as if to avoid an incoming attack. At the same time, paddle down the lower part of the cane in a counterclockwise curve to protect the outside of your right knee (Photo 20-1).

Movement 2

Stomp your right foot and rebound the energy from the floor to lift your left heel. At the same time, spin the cane on your right side with the tip up and handle hook down. Hold the cane vertically in front of the right side of your chest (Photo 20-2). Without stopping, step to the east with your left foot and shift weight to form a left-weighted, half-horseback-riding stance. Push the vertical cane toward the southeast corner (Photo 20-3).

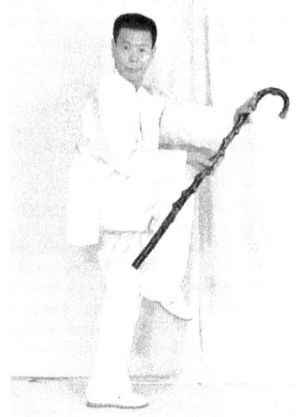

Photo 20-1

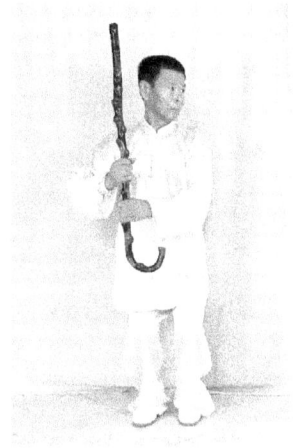

Photo 20-2

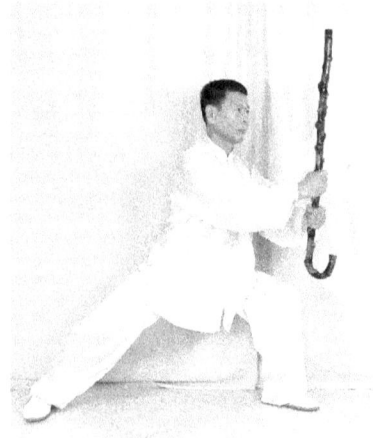

Photo 20-3

Movement 3

Spin the cane in front of your chest with the right hand leading the tail down and with your left hand flip the handle hook up. Hold the cane with your right hand about twelve inches away from the hook so the hook can be flipped up from the inner side of your right forearm (Photo 20-4).

Movement 4

Continue to spin the cane in your right hand counterclockwise until the cane is horizontal in front of your chest with the left palm touching your right wrist area to form a round bracing position (Photo 20-5). Next, strike the cane hook and left elbow sideways, still keeping your forearms rounded (Photo 20-6).

Key Points

1) Spin the cane two times counterclockwise. Make sure the spins are vertical in front of your torso for protection.

2) Your left toes should point halfway inward to the southeast corner to form the half-horseback-riding stance.

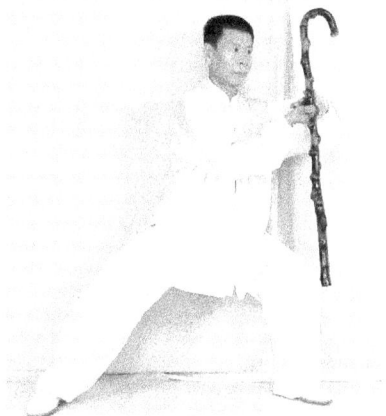

Photo 20-4

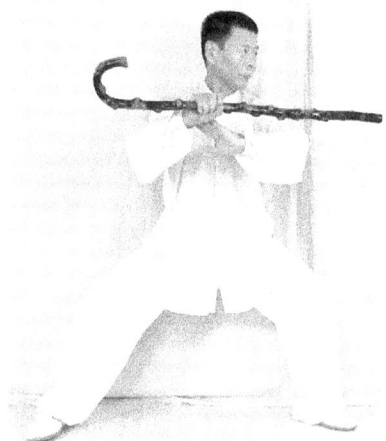

Photo 20-5

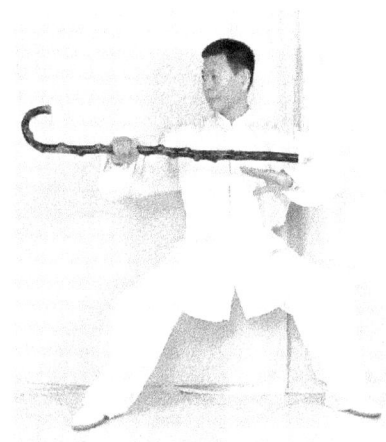

Photo 20-6

Posture 21: Single Whip 單鞭

Movement 1

Drop the cane tail slightly and push to your left side, then lift the cane above your head as if preparing to intercept an incoming weapon targeting your head. At the same time, drop your left elbow and lower your left palm to your right rib side (Photo 21-1).

Movement 2

Shift weight to your left foot to bend the left knee and stretch your right leg to form a left bow stance. At the same time, push your left palm to the east and raise the cane higher above your head with the hook end higher than the tip. Look to the east (Photo 21-2).

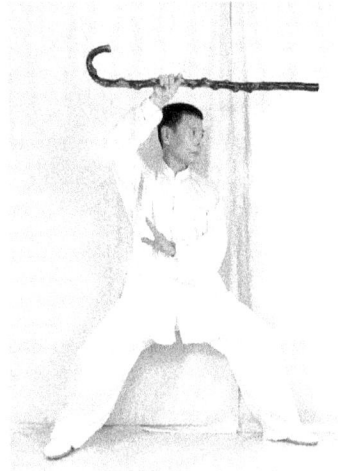

Photo 21-1

Key Points

1) This is a popular tai chi posture with the back leg powering your left palm to strike out. Use the cane to adhere to your opponent's weapon and redirect it upward. Immediately step forward with your left foot to close the distance and strike him with your left hand.

2) At the end, the cane acts as a bracing tool and balances the power of your palm strike to achieve your own energy harmony.

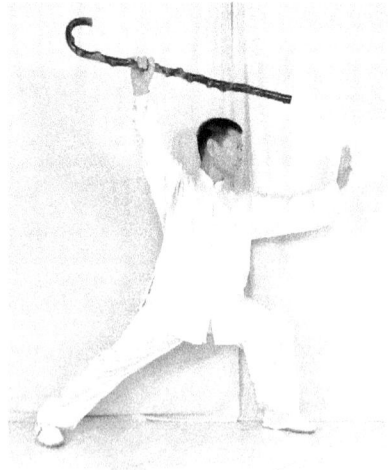

Photo 21-2

Posture 22: Cloud Hands 雲手

Movement 1

Shift weight to your right foot and wave the cane to your right side with the hook dropping down. Let the cane tail curve in a rainbow across your head from the east to the west side. At the same time, drop your left palm in front of your belly (Photo 22-1).

Movement 2

Continue to move the cane in a clockwise circle downward to line up with your right leg. At the same time, move your left palm in a counterclockwise circle up across your chest to your left side reaching face height (Photo 22-2). Without stopping, continue to circle your left palm down to your left side and circle your right hand up with the cane in front of your torso as you bring your right foot close to your left foot (Photo 22-3).

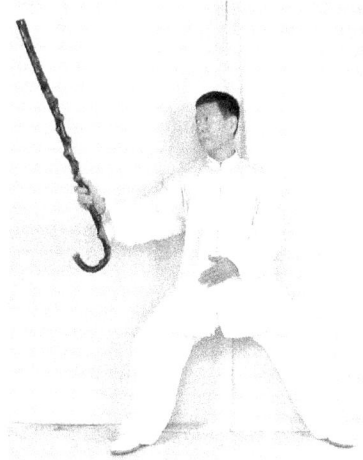

Photo 22-1

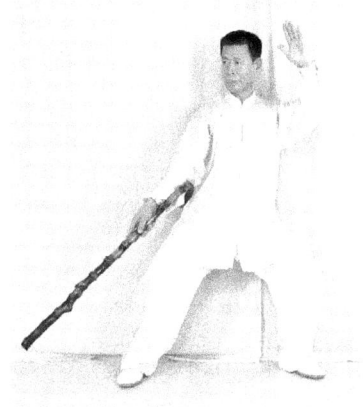

Photo 22-2

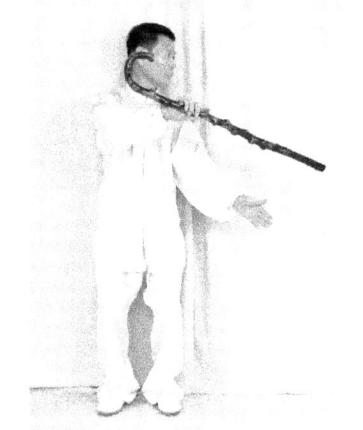

Photo 22-3

Movement 3

Wave the cane to your right in the same clockwise circle across the front of your head and move your left palm in the same counterclockwise circle in front of your belly (Photo 22-4).

Movement 4

Step your left foot to the left side as you wave the cane downward to your right and move your left hand up in front of your chest (Photo 22-5). Continue to move your left palm in the same counterclockwise circle down to the left side and move the cane in the clockwise circle up. At the same time, step your right foot close to the left foot (Photo 22-6).

Repeat the same moves as Movement 3 and 4 at least one more time, and, if the space allows, repeat a few more times.

Key Points

1) Cloud Hands is a popular tai chi posture with hands waving high outward and low inward in front of the torso. The cane is in your right hand as your right arm's extension. Your hands alternate high and low in harmony. When your hands are waving to your left side, your right foot steps in; when your hands are waving to the right side, your left foot steps out.

2) Use your torso's turning to initiate the motion of the arms.

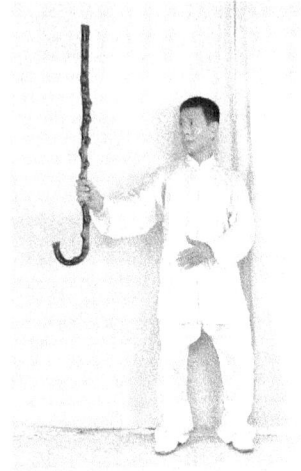

Photo 22-4

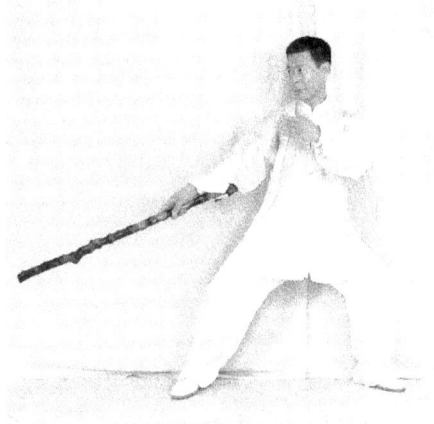

Photo 22-5

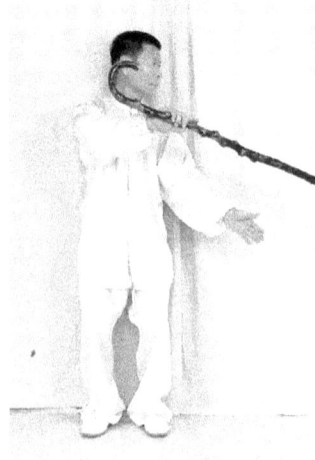

Photo 22-6

Posture 23: Single Whip 單鞭

Movement 1

Wave the cane to your right front and curve your left palm in front of your belly (Photo 23-1). Twirl your right wrist to lead the cane tail into a small counterclockwise circle and hold the cane in a horizontal position above your head. At the same time, shift weight to your right foot in a left empty stance with the ball of the left foot touching the floor. Your right palm faces out (Photo 23-2).

Movement 2

Step to the east with your left foot, bend the left knee, and stretch your right leg to form a left bow stance. At the same time, push your left palm to the east and brace the cane up to protect your head. Look to the east (Photo 23-3).

Key Point

This begins the same as Posture 21 but a small swirling circle changes the cane direction back to point to the east.

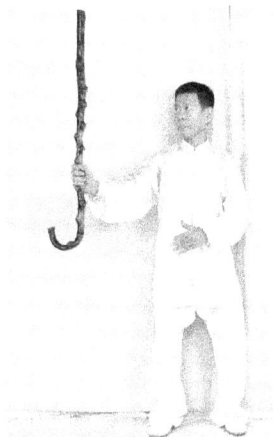

Photo 23-1

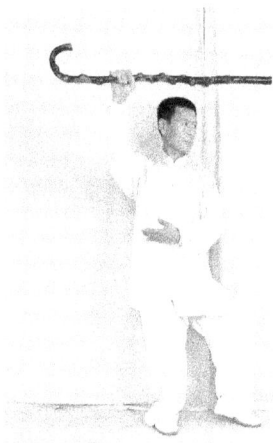

Photo 23-2

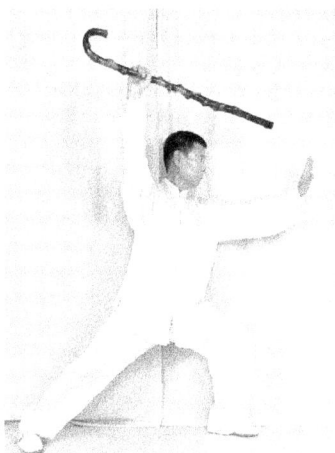

Photo 23-3

Posture 24: White Snake Flicks Tongue 白蛇吐信

Movement 1
Shift weight back to your right foot and withdraw the left foot a half step back. At the same time, drop your right hand with the cane parrying down in front of your face horizontally. The cane guards in front of your chest with the tip pointing to the north. Your left arm is under the cane with your palm facing up (Photo 24-1).

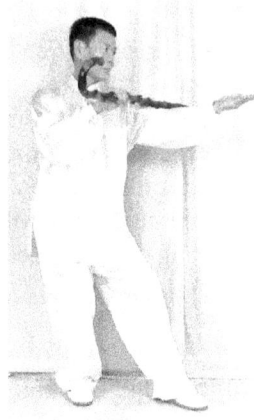

Movement 2
Push the cane out to guard your front and withdraw the left palm (Photo 24-2). Immediately step your left foot forward into a left bow stance and press the cane down. At the same time, thrust your left palm up above the cane to the east (Photo 24-3).

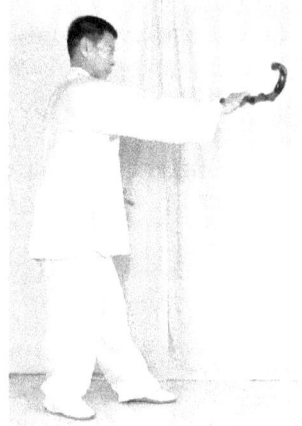

Key Points
1) Thrust your left palm under the cover of the cane.

2) Stretch your left fingers out to reach toward your opponent's eyes.

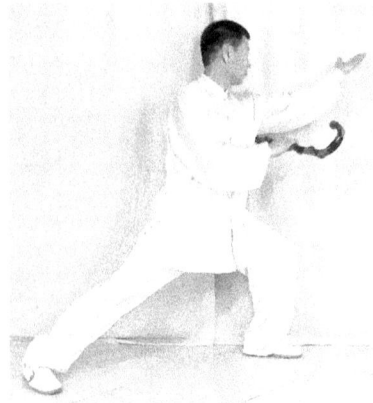

Photo 24-1

Photo 24-2

Photo 24-3

64

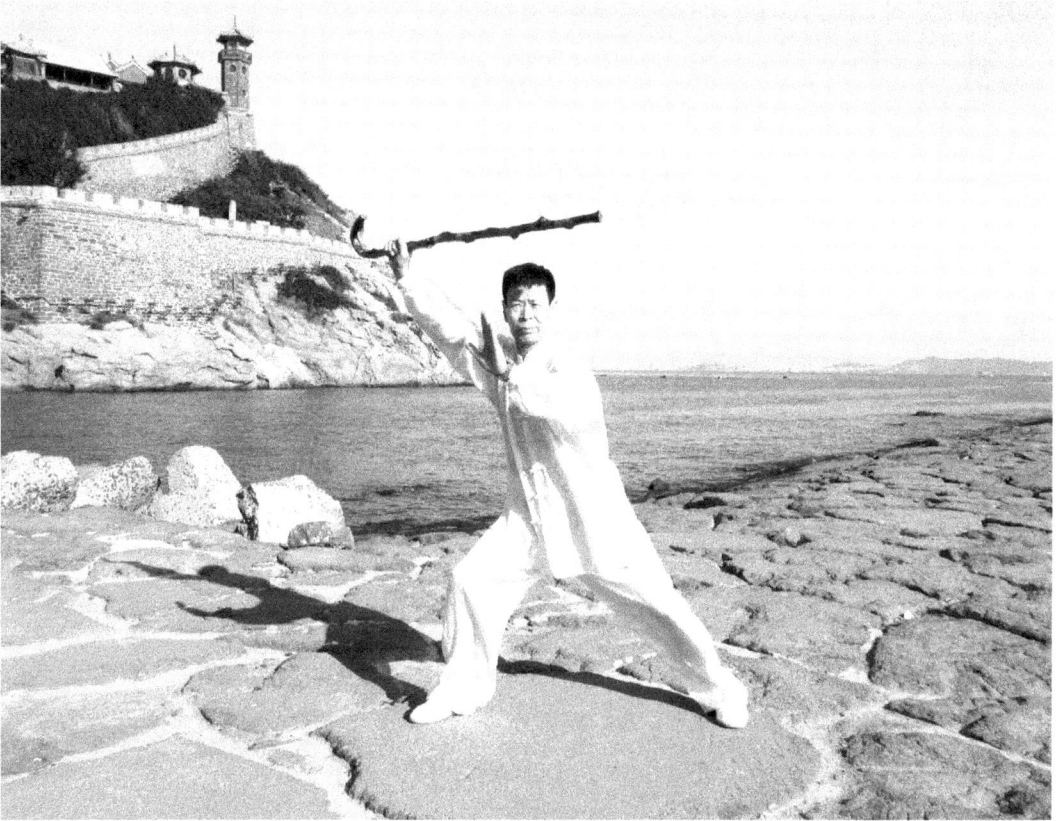

挑帘按掌

Flash Arms

Section IV

Posture 25: Crossover Hit 轉身十字杖

Movement 1

Shift your weight and turn the torso to your right to initiate the motion of sweeping the cane from your left side to the right. At the same time, close in your left forearm to ward off in front of your chest (Photo 25-1).

Movement 2

Continue the sweeping motion to whip the cane tail across your front to the right side (west) with your right arm extending straight and your left palm guarding in front of your chest. Sink your hips into a horseback riding stance (Photo 25-2).

Key Points

1) Use your torso's rotation to power the cane whipping to your right. You can shuffle your feet to support the right-side strike.

2) Optionally, you can move weight to your right foot to initiate the move and finish the strike with more weight on your left foot to balance the right-side hit.

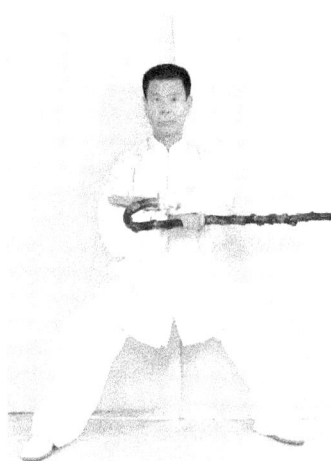

Photo 25-1

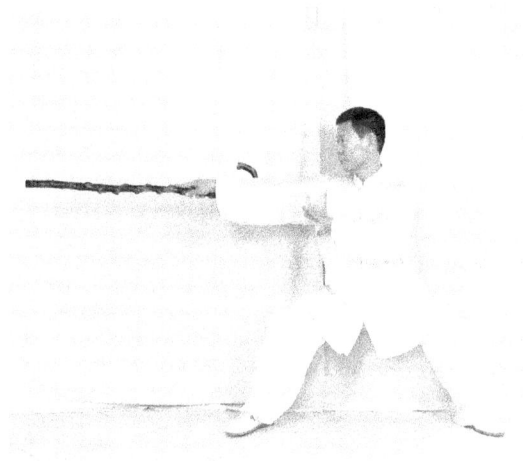

Photo 25-2

Posture 26: Push Boat Along the River 顺水推舟

Movement 1

Shift weight to your left foot and pull the right foot back. Parry the cane in an upper curve from the right to your left side as if you are deflecting an incoming weapon targeting your head. You can turn your left toes inward pointing to the south to facilitate the next move (Photo 26-1).

Movement 2

Circle the cane downward from the left side across your left leg. Step your right foot toward the west with a slight northwest angle into a right bow stance. At the same time, parry and push the cane in the direction of your right foot. The cane is diagonally in front of your torso with the hook side at head height (Photo 26-2).

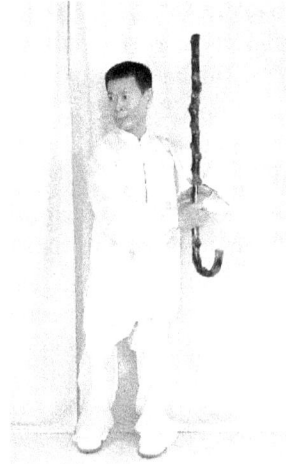

Photo 26-1

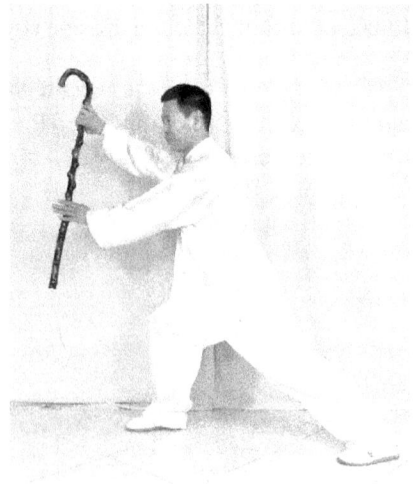

Photo 26-2

Movement 3

Seeming to pause without really pausing, go with the forward flow to follow up with your left foot in an empty stance, and hold the cane in the same position and pause momentarily. Maintain your hips sinking to keep the center of gravity low (Photo 26-3).

Movement 4

Shift weight onto your left foot and step your right foot back into a bow stance with the left leg bent at the knee. At the same time, maintain the cane in the same position bracing in front of your torso. These two movements are linked like an ocean wave flowing to shore and returning back to the ocean (Photo 26-4).

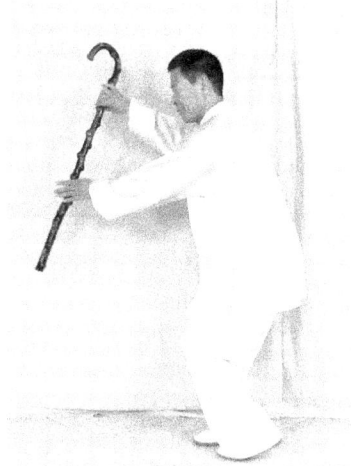

Photo 26-3

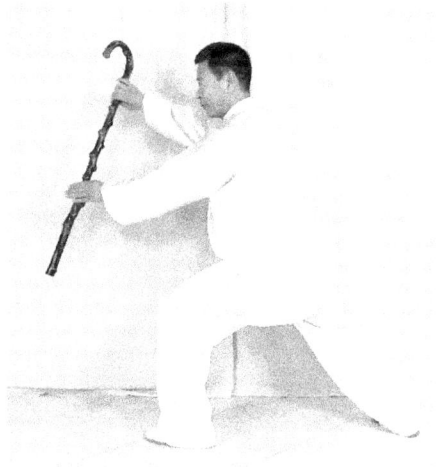

Photo 26-4

Movement 5

Shift weight back to your right foot and withdraw your left foot into a left empty stance again. At the same time, paddle the cane back alongside your left knee as if to parry away an incoming weapon targeting your left knee. Pause momentarily (Photo 26-5).

Movement 6

Step your left foot out into a left bow stance as you push the cane to the west. Feel the flow like ocean waves rushing to the shore. Hold the cane diagonally in front of your torso with the hook side up above your head (Photo 26-6).

Key Points

1) This posture trains your flexible stepping. When you step forward, the other foot follows up; when you step back, the other foot withdraws back.

2) Pay attention to the directions. Movement 2 faces a little bit northwest and Movement 6 faces directly to the west.

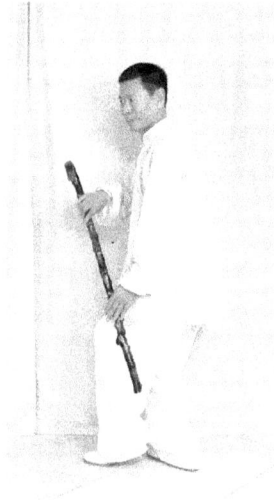

Photo 26-5

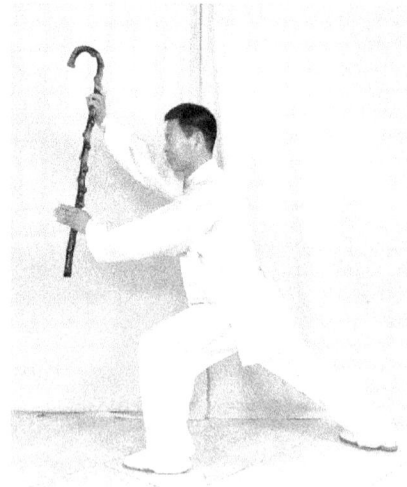

Photo 26-6

Posture 27: Circle the Lasso 雲杖斬击

Movement 1

Parry the cane to your left and circle it from your back, then circle it flat above your head as if you are lassoing a horse. Keep your left palm around your right wrist for support (Photo 27-1).

Movement 2

Lift your right knee up with the cane guarding in front of your head and ward off your left arm in front of your chest (Photo 27-2). Pause for a moment and then step forward with your right foot and circle the cane horizontally again before striking out. Bend your right knee into a right bow stance and stretch your left arm behind you (Photo 27-3).

Key Points

1) The lasso circle deflects an attack to your head. The second circle builds momentum for the strike.

2) You can hop on your left foot to gain distance to the west for the strike.

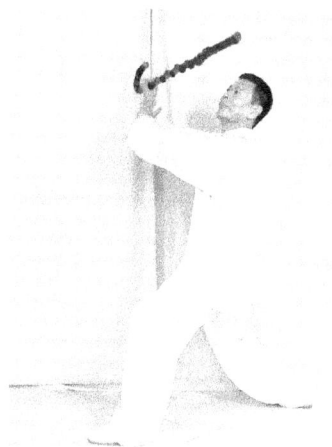
Photo 27-1

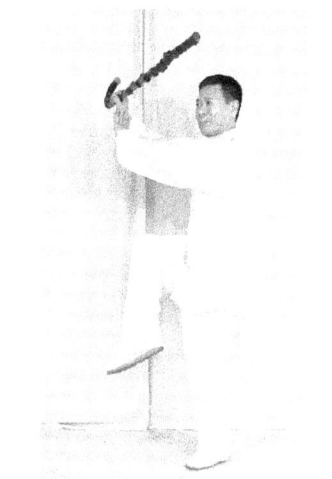
Photo 27-2

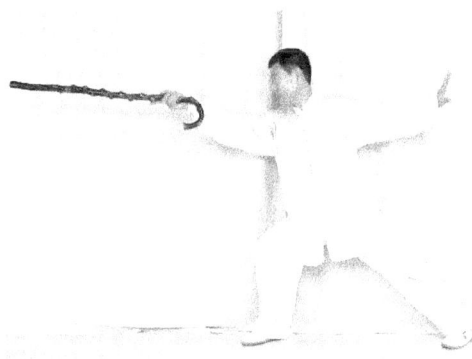
Photo 27-3

71

Posture 28: Flash Arms 挑帘推掌

Movement 1

Draw your right foot back with the ball of the foot touching the floor lightly and deflect the cane toward the left with the cane held diagonally in front of your face. Hold the cane with your right hand with palm facing your left chest and your left palm facing out supporting your right hand (Photo 28-1).

Movement 2

Circle the cane down to the left across your left leg and swing it up to the right. At the same time, turn your torso and step to the right (west) with the right foot and into a bow stance. The cane points to the west side with the tail at chest height and the handle above your head with the right palm facing out and the left palm supporting the right wrist area (Photo 28-2).

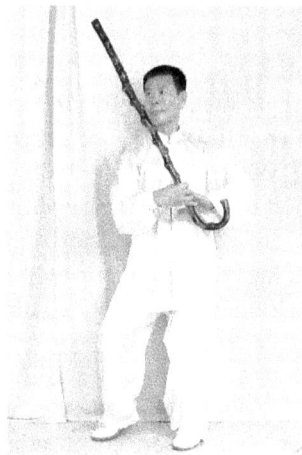

Photo 28-1

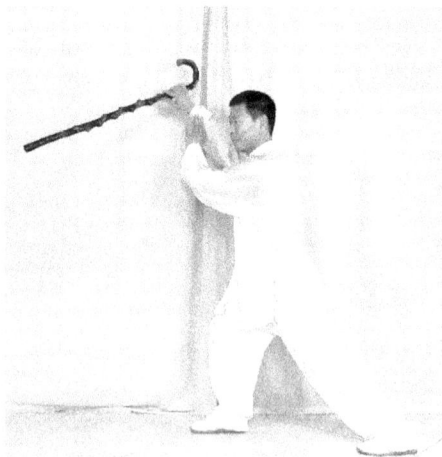

Photo 28-2

Movement 3

Lift and parry the cane tail to the right side of your head as if you are deflecting an incoming weapon targeting your head. At the same time, step to the west with your left foot while your left palm still guards in front of your chest. Keep the weight on the right leg (Photo 28-3).

Movement 4

Shift weight forward to your left foot and move into a left bow stance. At the same time, push your left palm to the west. At the end of this move, hold the cane with the tip a little lower than the hook but still higher than your head (Photo 28-4).

Key Points

1) These four moves are linked together with one circular swing of the cane. Your left step is under the protection of the circling cane, then strike with your left palm.

2) The left palm pushes to the west with fingers pointing up at your nose height. Your left arm should curve down slightly at the elbow but the arm itself lines up with your right leg.

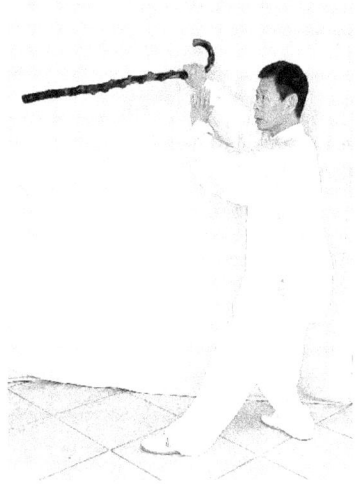

Photo 28-3

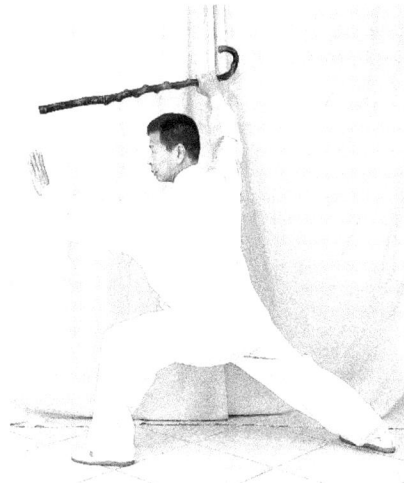

Photo 28-4

Posture 29: Whacking Strikes 迎风掸尘

Movement 1

Shift weight to your right foot and draw your left foot back a half step. Lower the cane handle from your upper front right corner in a clockwise curve with the cane held diagonally in front of your chest. Cautiously look to the front (Photo 29-1).

Movement 2

Step forward and a little to the left southwest corner with your left foot, swirl the cane tip clockwise in a tiny circle, whack the cane to your left front (southwest corner), and move into a left bow stance. Your hands should hold the cane handle in front of your left shoulder with the tip of the cane above your head. Look at the tip (Photo 29-2).

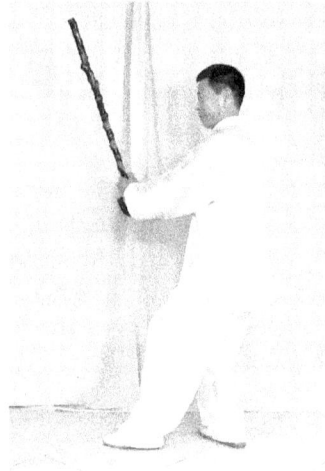

Photo 29-1

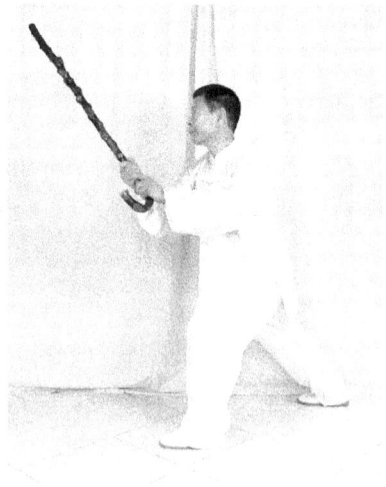

Photo 29-2

Movement 3

Turn your torso a little to the left and pull your right foot close to the left. At the same time, swirl the cane tip counterclockwise in a tiny circle and hold the cane guarding your front left chest. The tiny circle is a result of your torso's twist to the left. You don't have to make a small circle at the tip if it is difficult. Look at the tip of the cane (Photo 29-3).

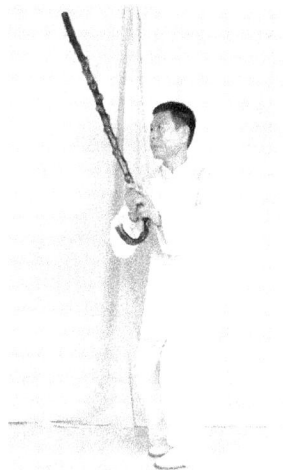

Movement 4

Seeming to pause without really pausing, immediately step forward a little to the right side (northwest corner) with your right foot, then whack the cane to your right front toward the northwest. Bend your right knee into a right bow stance. Hold the cane handle in front of your right shoulder and look at the cane tip (Photo 29-4).

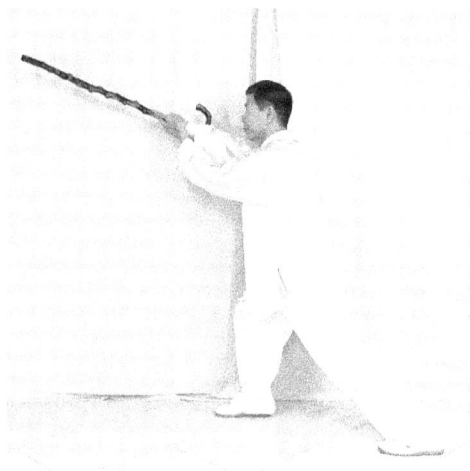

Photo 29-3

Photo 29-4

Movement 5

Turn your torso a little to the right and pull your left foot close to the right foot with the left heel off the floor. At the same time, swirl the cane tip clockwise in a tiny circle and hold the cane guarding your front right chest (Photo 29-5).

Movement 6

Seeming to pause without really pausing, immediately step forward a little to the left side (southwest corner) with your left foot and bend your left knee into a bow stance. At the same time, whack the cane to the left front. Your hands should hold the cane handle in front of your left shoulder as you look at the cane tip (Photos 29-5 and 29-6).

Key Points

1) This posture links three strikes toward your opponent's head and is based on the traditional Yang tai chi sword technique.

2) As you reach the advanced level, make sure there is a tiny swirling circle so the cane can smoothly reverse the striking direction.

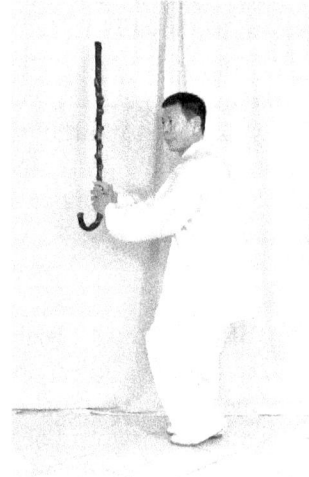

Photo 29-5

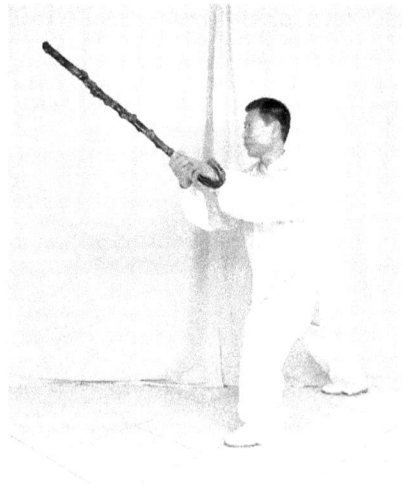

Photo 29-6

Posture 30: Cat Pounces on Mouse 靈猫撲鼠

Movement 1

Maintaining the cane in a ward-off left position, slide the cane to your left rib side, and at the same time kick your right foot forward. Imagine you are keeping the cane in continuous contact with your opponent's weapon (Photo 30-1).

Movement 2

Lower your right foot and return it to the same spot at your right rear. At the same time, thrust the cane out from your left rib side with the tip pointed to the opponent's face (Photo 30-2). Pay attention that your stance is the same as in Photo 29-6, but your hands' and the cane's function are totally different.

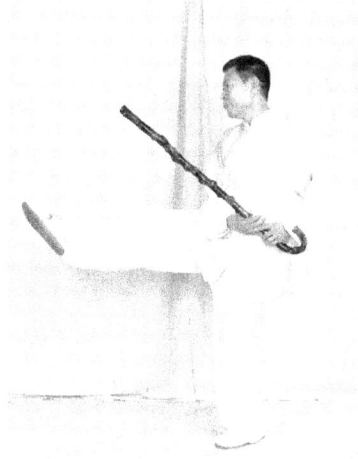

Photo 30-1

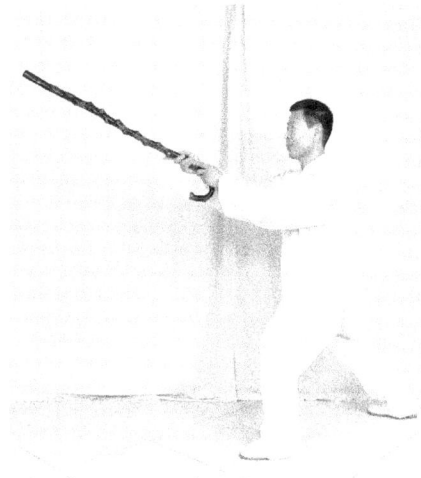

Photo 30-2

Movement 3

Drop the cane tip and twirl your right wrist to circle the cane vertically outside your right arm. At the same time, withdraw the left foot halfway back (Photo 30-3).

Movement 4

Immediately peck the cane tip toward the floor with your left palm pressed at the middle of the cane. Lift the handle end up with the right hand, and bend your torso at the waist (Photo 30-4).

Key Points

1) Make sure the cane continues contact with an incoming weapon to cover your right foot's kick out.

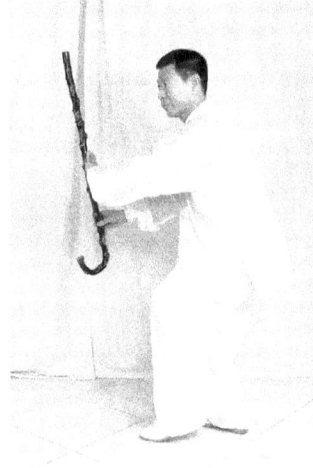

Photo 30-3

2) When you return the right foot back, you can use a small, quick, backward jump and strike the cane tip downward in front of you.

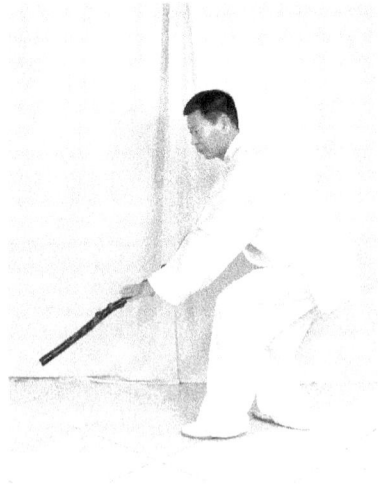

Photo 30-4

Posture 31: *Taming Tiger* 左右打虎篦式

Movement 1

Point the cane tail up in front of you and parry the cane in an upper curve to your left side with the left hand on top. At the same time, step toward the southwest corner with your left foot (Photo 31-1).

Movement 2

Turn your torso to the left and bend your left knee into a left bow stance. At the same time, continue to parry the cane to the left front. Keep both arms rounded out to brace the cane strongly (Photo 31-2).

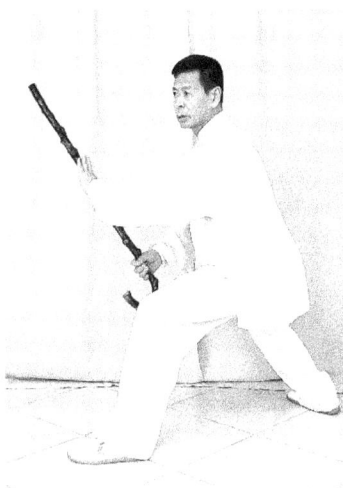

Photo 31-1

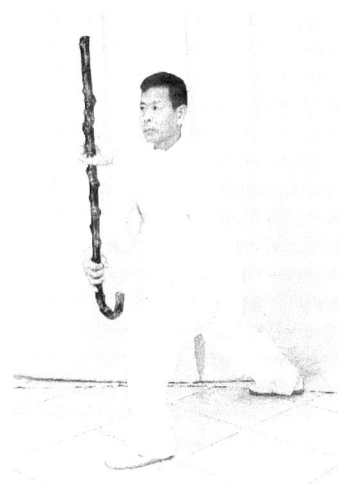

Photo 31-2

Movement 3

Pull your right foot in toward the left foot, and at the same time, spin the cane counterclockwise with the right hand hook end on top. Hold the cane a little closer to your chest for protection (Photo 31-3).

Movement 4

Step toward the northwest corner with your right foot, bend your right knee, and stretch the left leg into a bow stance. At the same time, continue to parry the cane to the right front. Look to the west (Photo 31-4).

Key Points

1) This move is rooted in the traditional Yang tai chi barehand form. Here you use the cane as a shield to protect your left and right.

2) Make sure to use your torso's turning to power the cane's move.

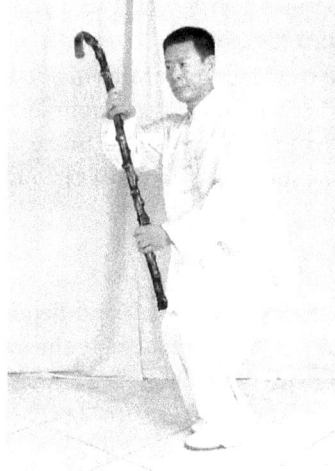

Photo 31-3

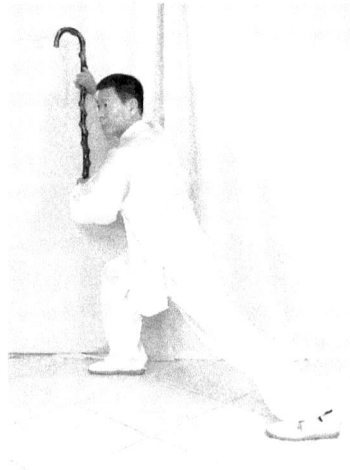

Photo 31-4

Posture 32: Cane Whacks Head 當頭杖

Movement 1
Shift weight to the left leg almost into a horseback riding stance, and turn your torso to lead the cane parry to your left side. Continue to hold the cane vertically with your right hand on top and left hand at the bottom. Look to the east (Photo 32-1).

Movement 2
Slide your left hand up to meet the right hand near the hook, and wrap the cane from the outside of your left arm across your back to the back of your right shoulder. Keep the cane relatively vertical behind you (Photo 32-2).

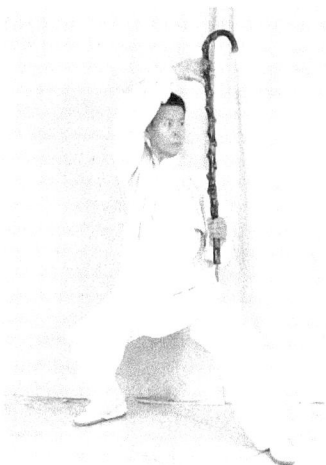

Photo 32-1

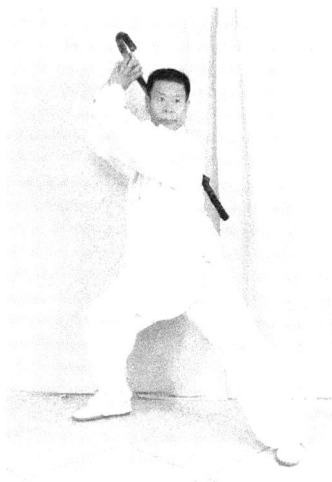

Photo 32-2

Movement 3

Drop the cane from outside your right arm and sweep it horizontally across your front to the left side. Relax both wrists at the end of the sweep to allow the cane to land softly on the outside of your left arm. Your eyes follow the cane to the east. Still remain in a firm horseback riding stance (Photo 32-3).

Movement 4

Sweep the cane from your left side horizontally across your front to the right side. Relax both wrists at the end of the sweep to allow the cane to land softly on the outside of your left arm. Still hold a firm horseback riding stance. Your eyes follow the cane to the west (Photo 32-4).

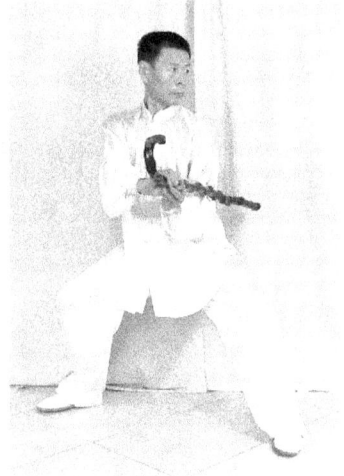

Photo 32-3

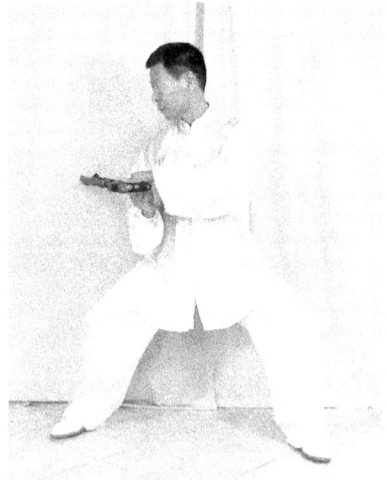

Photo 32-4

Movement 5

Twist your arms from your right shoulder side to raise your hands above your head and hold the cane vertically behind your back. You are still in the horseback riding stance (Photo 32-5). Immediately hack the cane from behind to your front with the cane lined up with your arms at shoulder height. You are still in the horseback riding stance facing the southwest corner (Photo 32-6).

Key Points

1) Wrapping the cane from front to back and sweeping left and right are all driven by your torso's turning. Maintain a strong horseback riding stance to power these moves.

2) Extend your arms and let the power reach to the front of the cane when hacking down to the front.

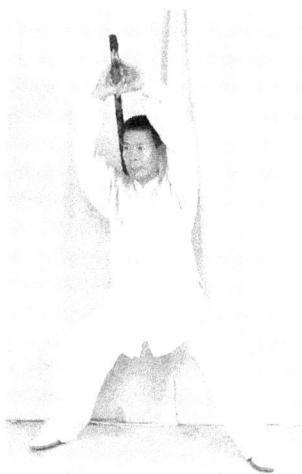

Photo 32-5

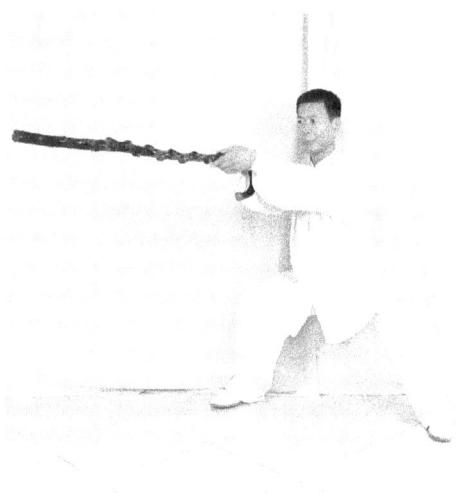

Photo 32-6

Posture 33: White Tiger Sweeps Tail 白篦摆尾

Movement 1

Parry the cane above your head horizontally for protection and shift weight to your right foot. At the same time, push the left palm in front of your chest to the southwest corner (Photo 33-1).

Movement 2

Lower the cane tail and hold it vertically while parrying to your left side. At the same time, step the left foot across the front of your right leg to the west into a cross stance, with your left palm moving to your right rib side as you look to your left side (Photo 33-2).

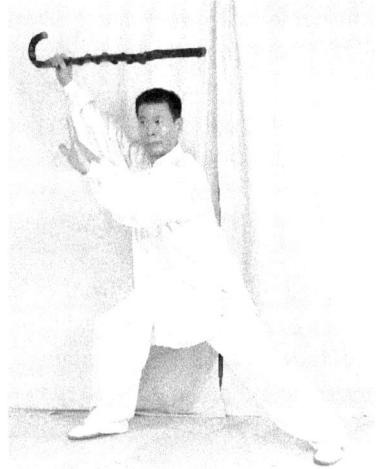

Photo 33-1

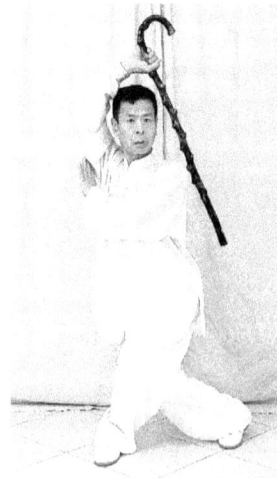

Photo 33-2

Movement 3

Step to the right (west) with your right foot and push the left palm to your left (east). At the same time, wrap the cane from outside your left shoulder to the back and hold the cane handle above your right shoulder. You are in a horseback riding stance with the cane behind your neck. Look to your left (Photo 33-3).

Movement 4

Sweep the cane from behind across the front of your torso horizontally until your right hand touches your left rib side with the cane tip pointing back. At the same time, close your left arm with the palm facing west touching your right upper arm (Photo 33-4). Immediately sweep the cane from your left side across your front to your right side. Bend your right wrist to let the cane rest on the back of your neck (Photo 33-5).

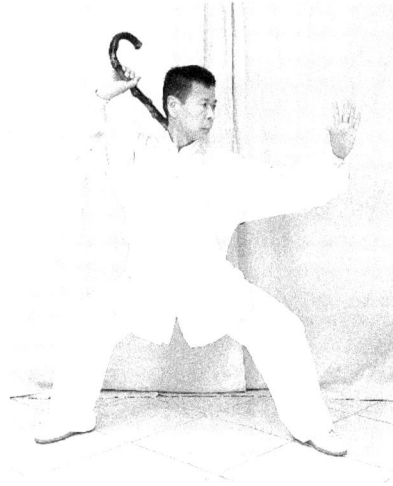

Photo 33-3

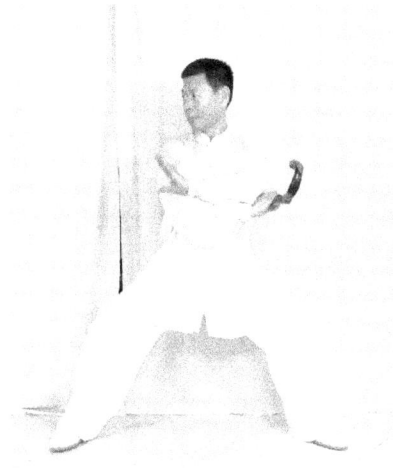

Photo 33-4

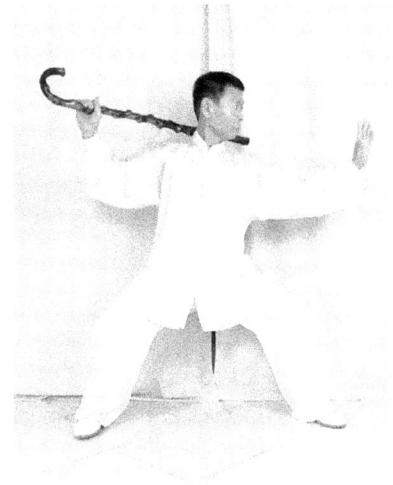

Photo 33-5

Movement 5

Pivoting on your left heel, turn the left toes outward and to the north and turn your torso to the left. Step to the east with the right foot into a horseback riding stance. Repeat Movement 4 but face the north (Photos 33-6 and 33-7).

Key Points

1) This posture is built on three close-open arm motions to sweep the cane around your torso. It is rooted in the Taoist whisk self-defense.

2) Remain in horseback riding stance to power the cane sweep as if it were a tiger's tail whipping around. The horseback riding stance provides a firm foundation for the sweeping motions of the arm and cane.

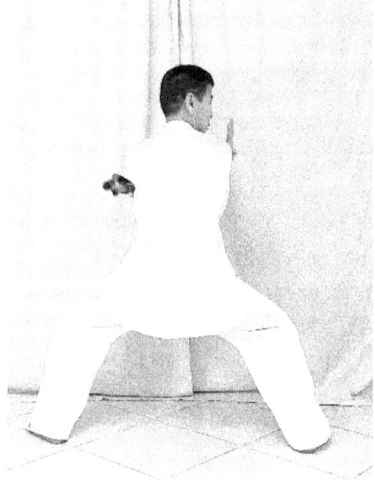

Photo 33-6

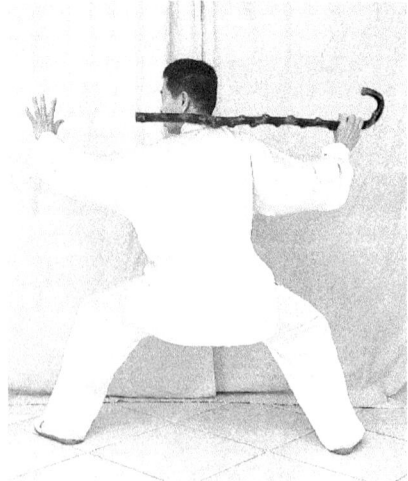

Photo 33-7

Posture 34: Cane Guards Heart 護心杖

Movement 1

Wrap the cane around your head from the back of your neck to move the cane handle in front of your chest with the cane above your left shoulder. Turn your torso to the left and draw the left palm in a curve down between the cane and your chest (Photo 34-1).

Movement 2

Pull the left foot halfway back into a left empty stance. Press your left palm at the middle of the cane to guard your heart with the cane tip pointing diagonally forward to the west (Photo 34-2).

Key Point

This is a simple protection pose using the cane to ward off incoming weapons.

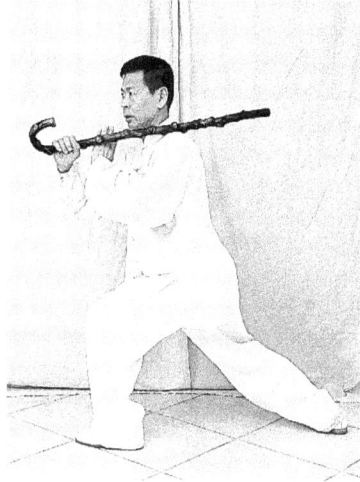

Photo 34-1

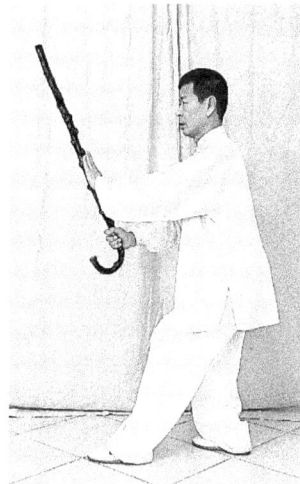

Photo 34-2

Posture 35: Immortal Points a Way Out 仙人指路

Movement 1
Lift your left knee and paddle the cane tip downward to protect in front of your left knee. Keep the left palm around the middle of the cane (Photo 35-1).

Movement 2
Spin the cane on your left side to flip the cane tail from the lower left to point to the west with your left palm touching at your right wrist. At the same time, lower your left foot with toes pointing to the southwest corner and both knees slightly bent (Photo 35-2).

Movement 3
Lift your right knee and stand upright on your left leg. Thrust the cane to the west and extend your left palm to the southeast corner (Photo 35-3).

Key Points
1) Deflect an incoming weapon and crouch to store up energy.

2) Thrust the cane out like a rattlesnake attacking its prey.

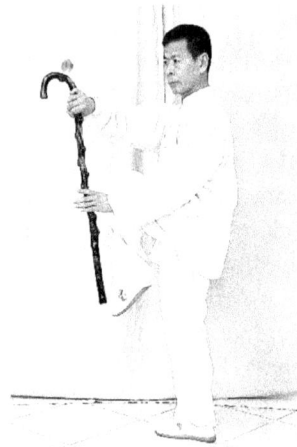
Photo 35-1

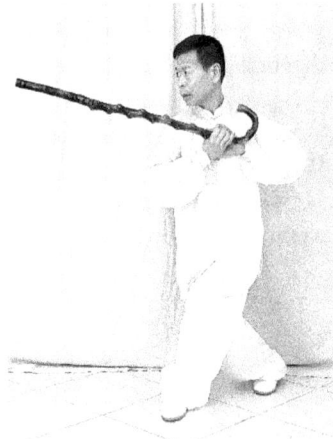
Photo 35-2

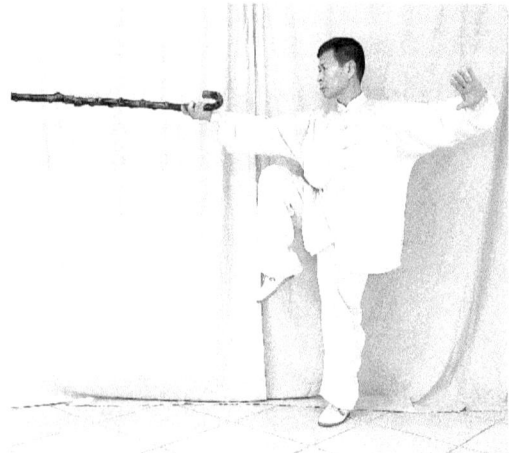
Photo 35-3

Posture 36 Closing Form 收势

Movement 1

Step in a big circle with your right foot, toes pointing outward. Turn your torso to the right with the cane parrying to your right side, and keep your left palm turned up to the left (Photo 36-1).

Movement 2

Continue the turn to your right with your left foot and step in an inward curve to drive your turn spin to your right. Keep the cane and left palm in the same position, and let your torso spin to sweep the cane in a large circle. You can take a few small steps to make the turn complete (Photo 36-2).

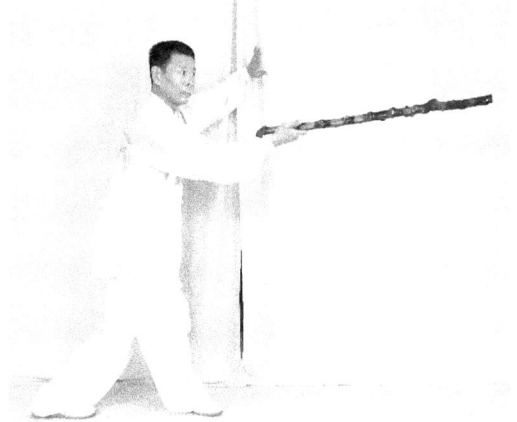

Photo 36-1

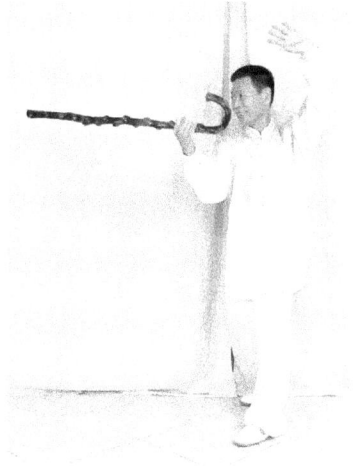

Photo 36-2

Movement 3

As you finish sweeping the cane in the large circle, close the left palm in and let the cane tail point down and then continue the cane movement into another small circle wrapping around your head. You will face the south at the end of the circle steps (Photo 36-3).

Movement 4

Step your right foot toward the right front corner (southwest, Photo 36-4) and land the cane tip a few inches in front of the right foot. At the same time, push your left palm toward the southeast corner (Photo 36-5).

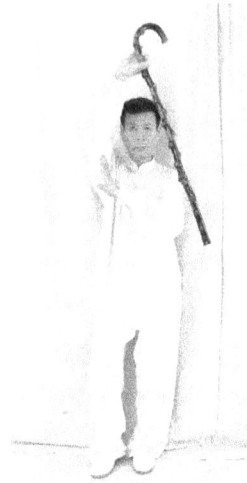

Photo 36-3

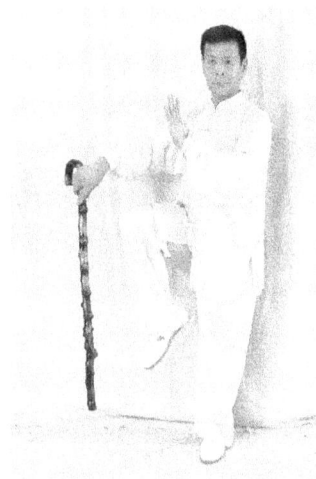

Photo 36-4

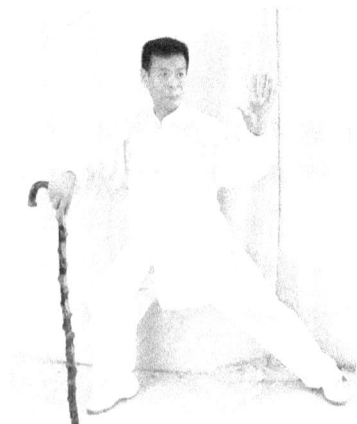

Photo 36-5

Movement 5

Step your left foot in so it is parallel with your right foot, keeping your feet about shoulder width apart. At the same time, return the left palm in an upper curve back in front of your chest with fingers pointing up like a prayer (Photo 36-6). Then drop the left palm down to the side of the left hip and close your left foot next to the right foot (Photo 36-7).

Key Points

1) The large circle sweeping the cane is driven by your circling steps and torso's spin. Keep the cane extended out as far as you can to clear your surroundings; the small circle wraps around your head to return energy back to your torso.

2) The left palm curves back in front of your chest and drops down as if silk reeling to coil energy back to your lower belly dantian.

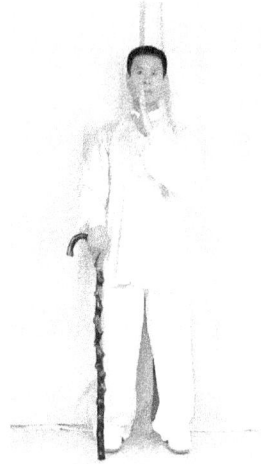

Photo 36-6

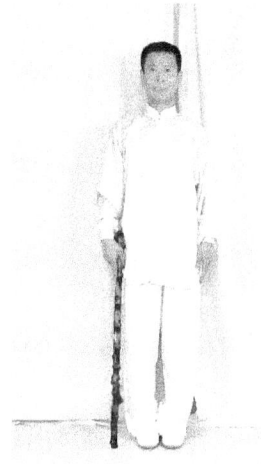

Photo 36-7

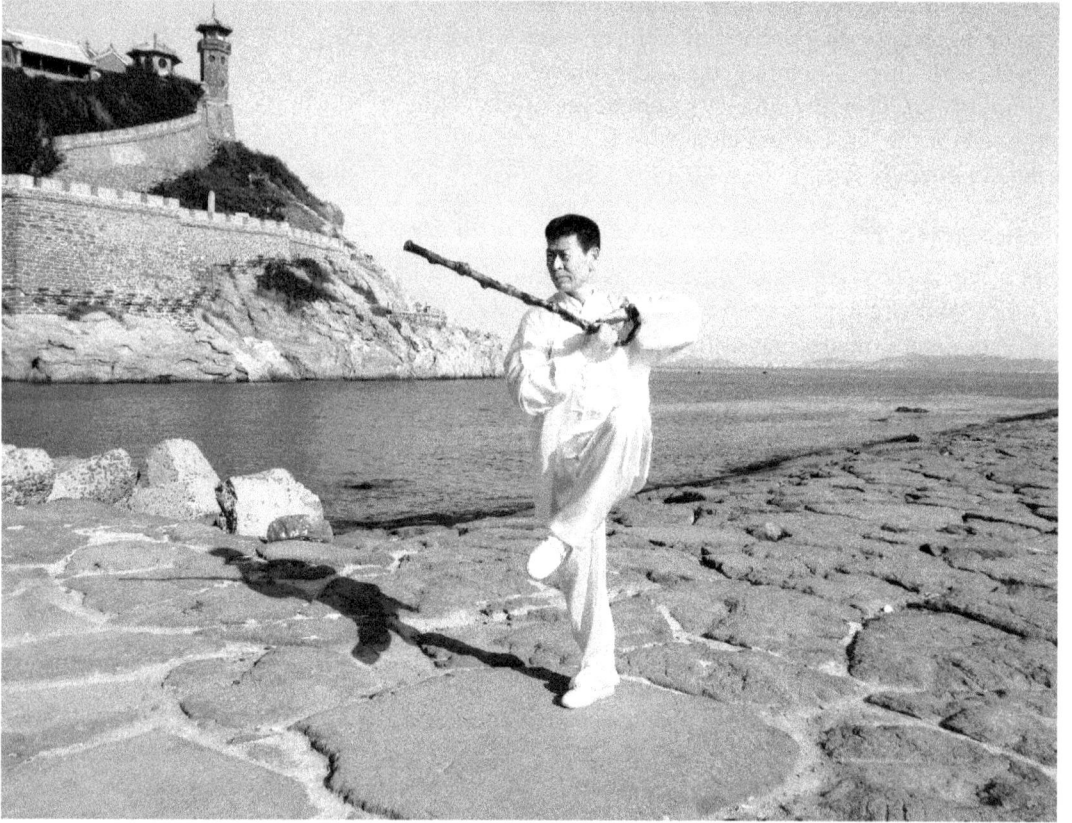

Section V

Photo series of Jesse Tsao practicing Eight-Immortals Tai Chi Cane in front of Penglai Temple where the Eight Immortals legend originated

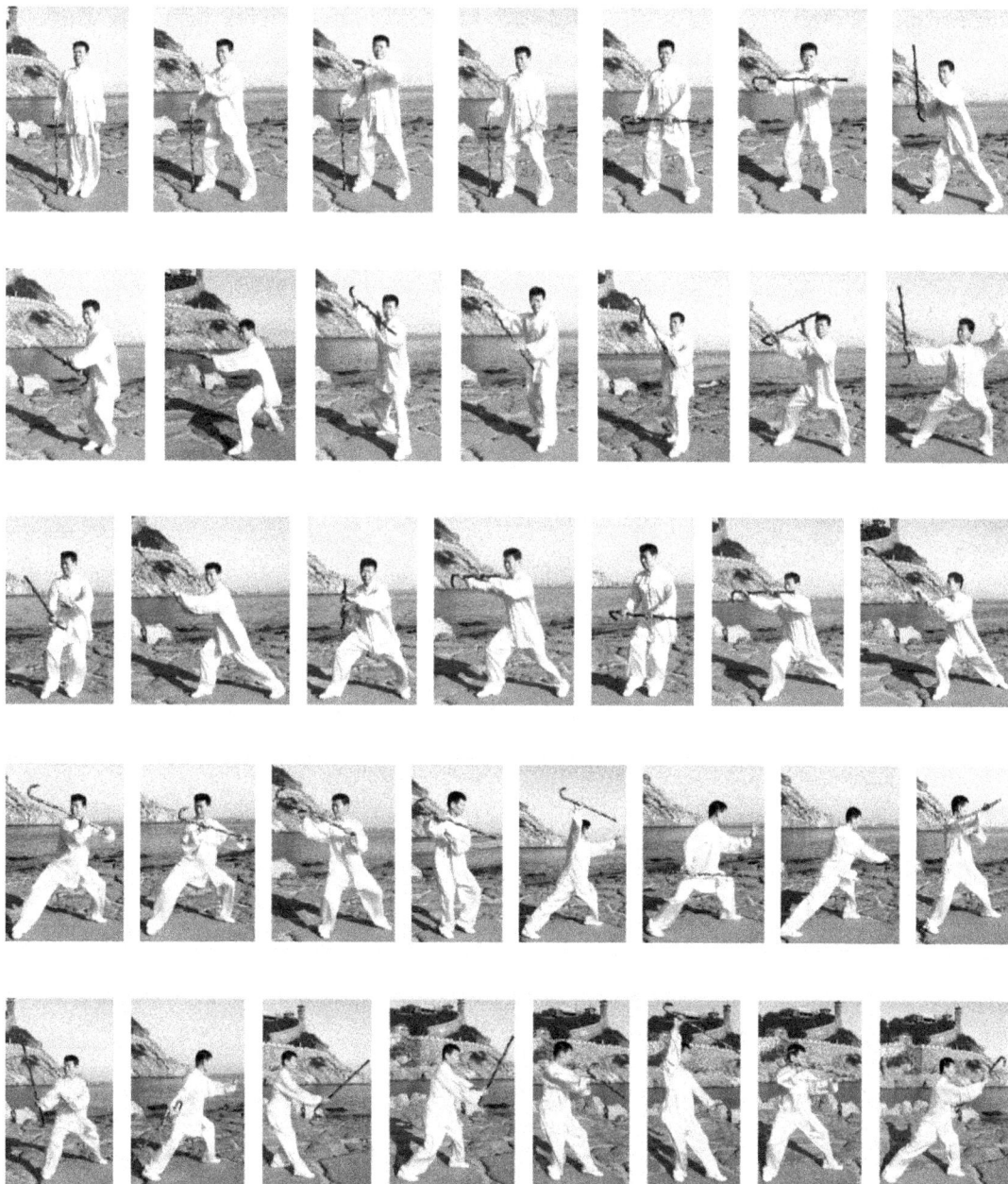

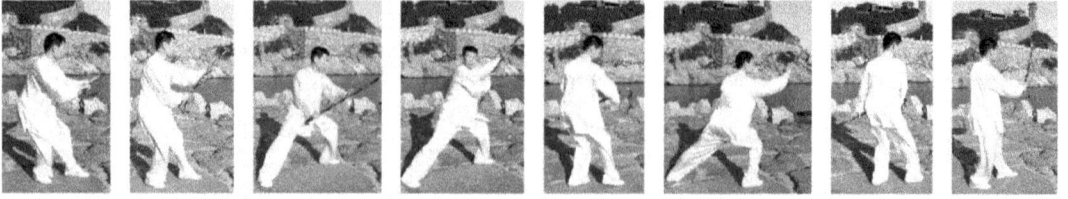

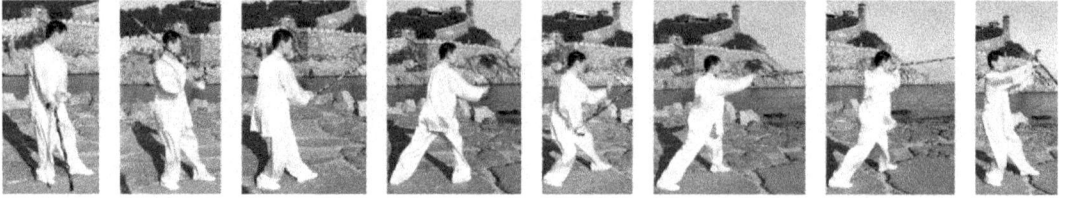

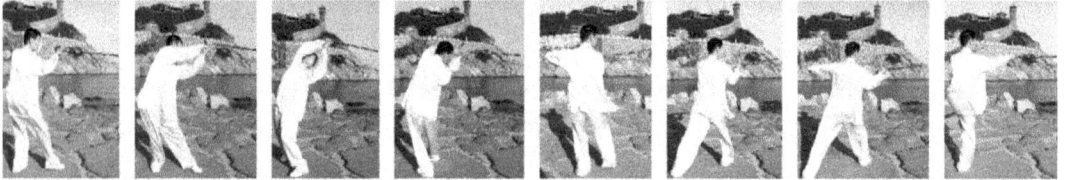

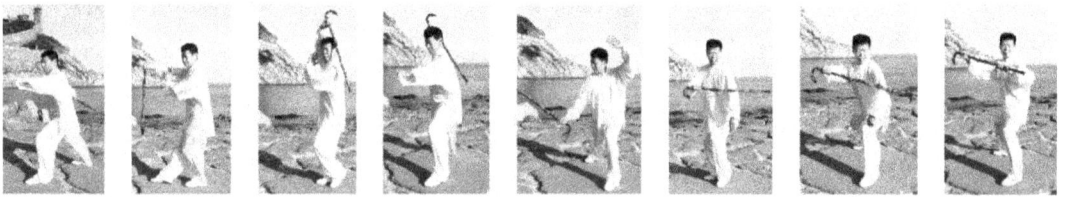

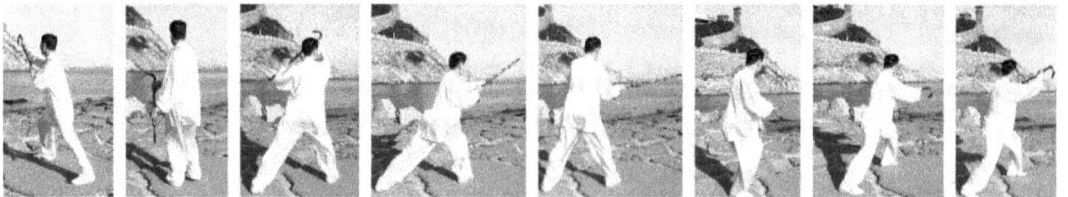

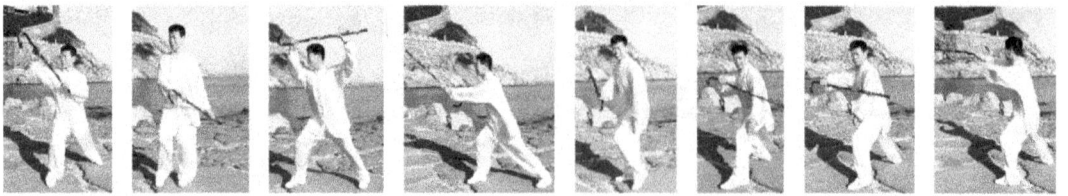

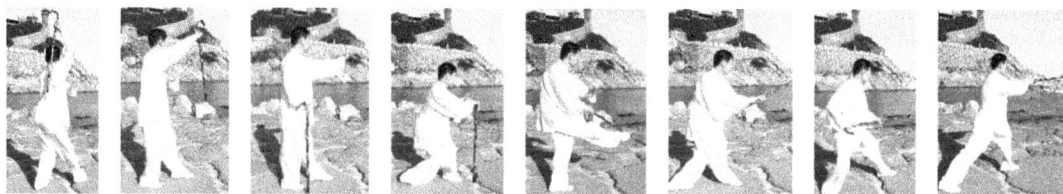

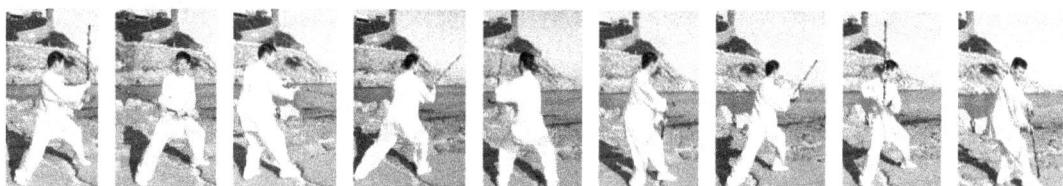

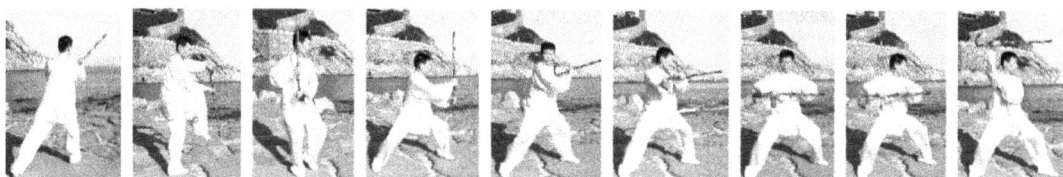

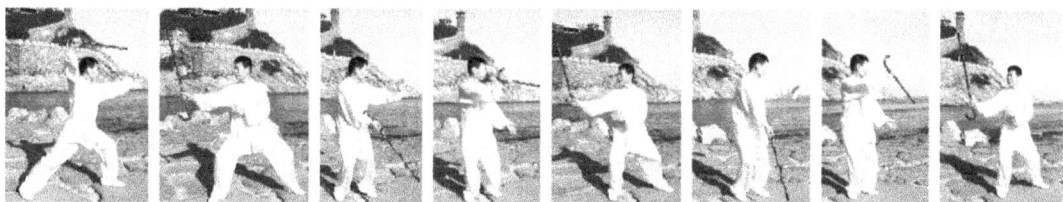

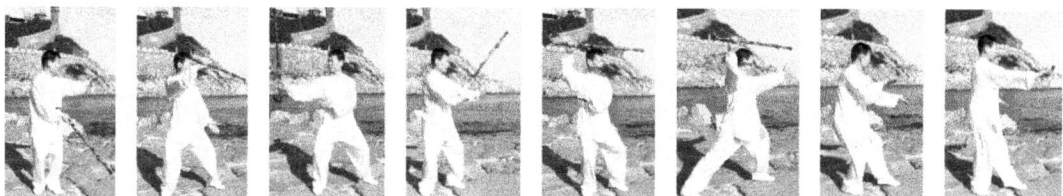

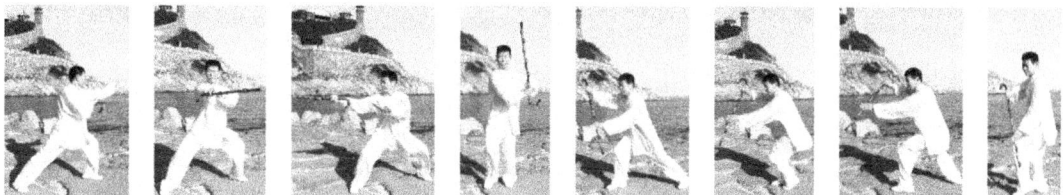

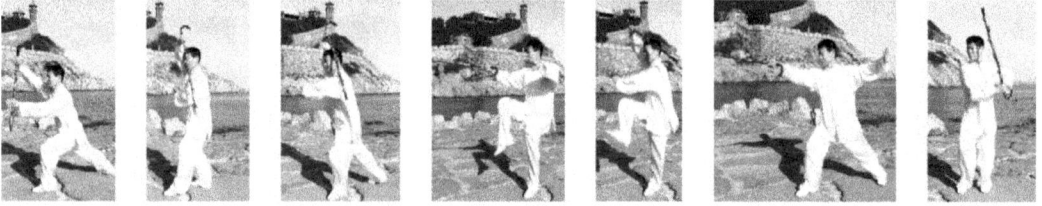

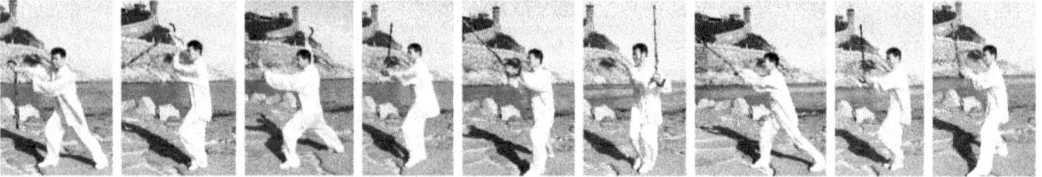

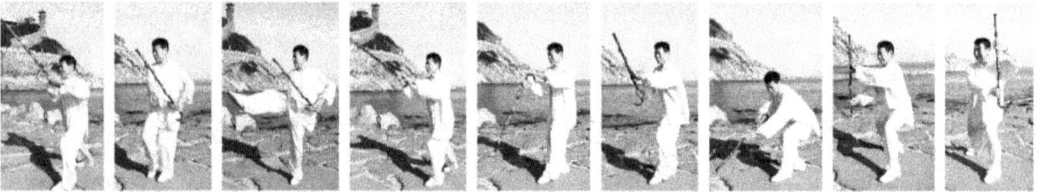

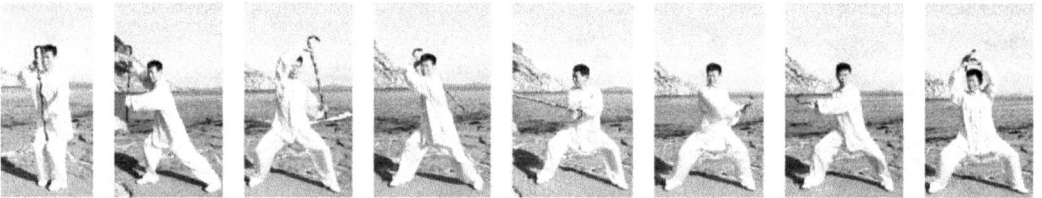

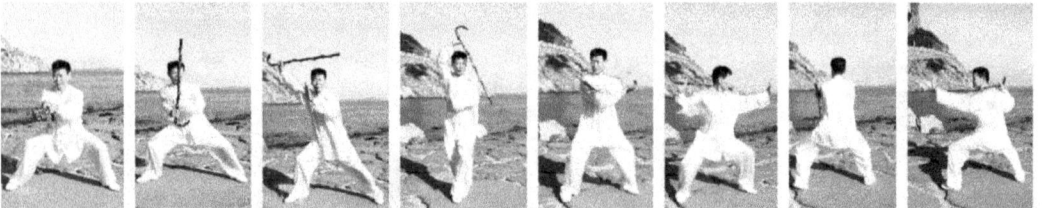

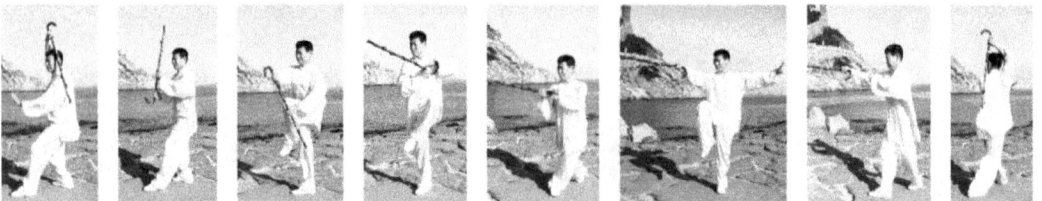

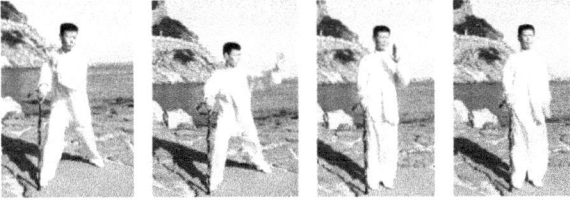

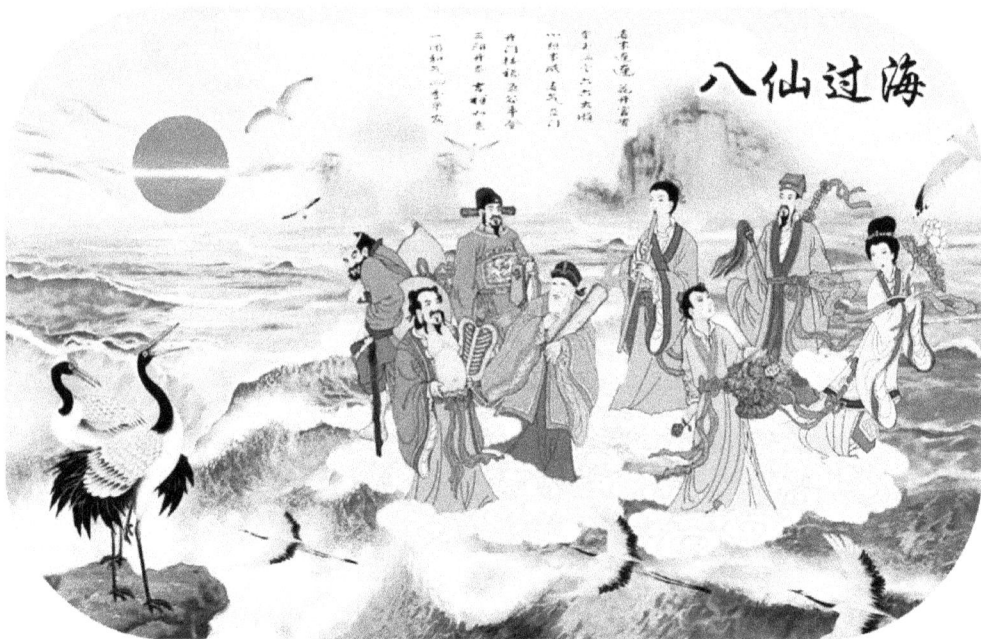

八仙過海

*Eight Immortals
Crossing the Sea*

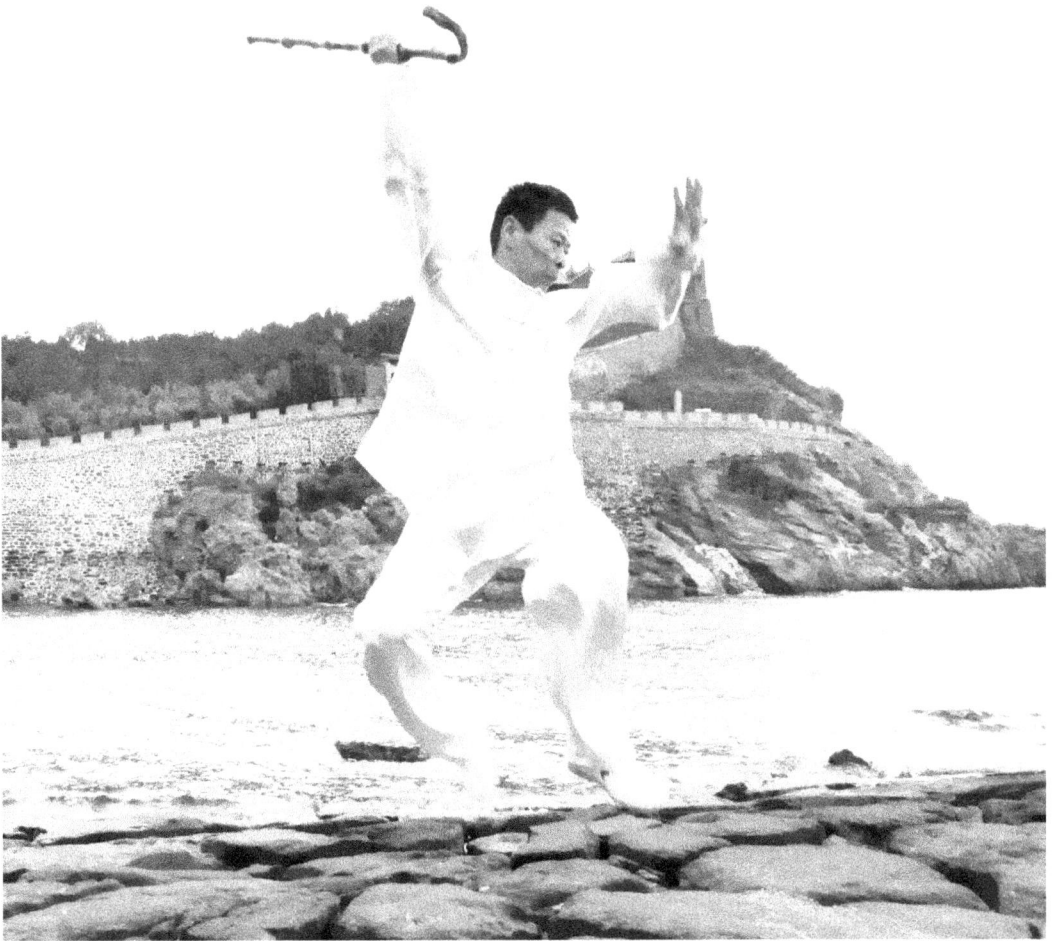

翻花舞袖

Whipping Sleeves & Slamming Cane

Part II
Traditional Tai Chi Eight-Immortals Cane Routine II (Based on Chen Style)

Routine II is the answer for people looking for the internal power of tai chi. Like the Chen-style tai chi cannon fist, this routine is packed with powerful moves and explosive strikes. Chen style is the oldest and considered to be the "parent" of the five major tai chi styles. It alternates between fast and slow movements combined together with jumping and stomping. Not only does this routine consist of exercises balanced between yin and yang, it also emphasizes the power moves to echo Yang style's soft approach in Routine I.

According to the philosophy of Taoism, everything is composed of two opposite elements of yin and yang working in a relationship that is in perpetual balance. Yin and yang are polar opposites and are found in all things in life. In nature, everything tends toward a natural state of harmony. Concepts such as dark, soft, pliant, yielding, and feminine are associated with yin, while concepts such as bright, hard, rigid, and masculine are associated with yang. Both sides complement each other and together form a perfect whole. Therefore, Routine II was created to complement Routine I. Things perfectly balanced and in harmony are at peace, and being at peace leads naturally to longevity.

Section 1

Posture 1: Opening Form 起勢

Movement 1

In preparation for Opening Form, stand relaxed with feet shoulder-width apart, loosen your waist, and unlock your hips to lower your center of gravity. Find your central equilibrium by containing your chest and lifting your spine as if an intangible energy rope lifts the crown of your head. Imagine there is a central axis passing through your torso from head to tailbone. Stay in this pose for a moment until you feel your spine elongate and the spaces between the vertebrae open. The cane is at the side of your right leg, near the right foot. Calm your mind and settle your breath deep into the lower abdomen (Photo 1-1).

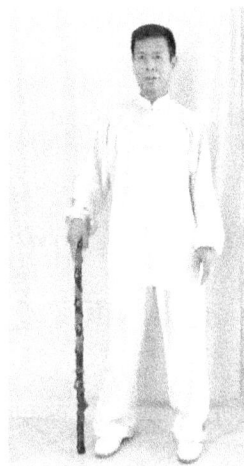

Photo 1-1

Movement 2

Purposely sink your left hip a little more and turn your torso to your right, chest facing the southwest corner. At the same time, sink your shoulders and circle your left hand up in front of your chest to chin height with palm facing toward your chest. Feel the peng (ward off) energy maintaining a space between your left arm and your chest (Photo 1-2).

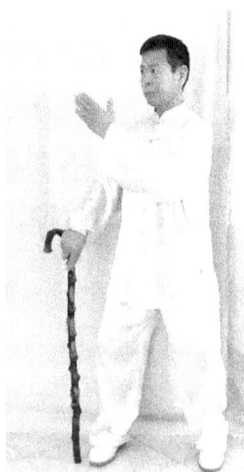

Photo 1-2

Movement 3

Turn your torso to the left and move your left palm in an upper curve outward toward the southeast front corner. At the same time, turn the left palm facing outward, eyes following your left palm (Photo 1-3).

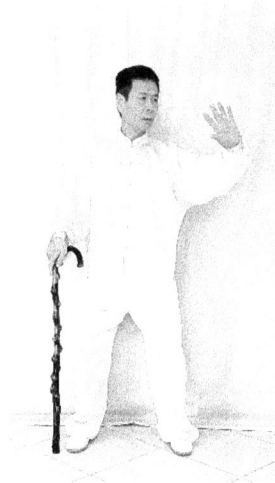

Photo 1-3

Movement 4

Circle your left palm downward and return it to the left side of your belly. Sink both hips a little more by bending both knees slightly and settle down your dantian (the center of your lower abdomen) with a deep exhale. This movement will create a gentle outward pressure on your inner thighs and you should feel the crotch (the space between your inner thighs) rounding as an arched stone bridge. The ward-off energy of your pelvis enables you to hold your torso in a stable position (Photo 1-4).

Key Points

1) If possible, face the south to start the form with your left side to the east and your right side to the west. The directions that follow assume you began the form facing the south.

2) In preparation, relax the mind and body to allow your inner energy to circulate without blockage.

3) Sink your left hip to get the earth rebound energy for your dantian rotation to give birth to the silk reeling of your left hand. Let your torso motion lead your arm and hand.

4) Unlock and sink your hips to round your crotch at the end in preparation for the next move.

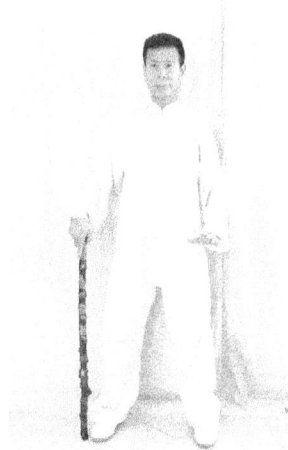

Photo 1-4

Posture 2: Lazily Tying Coat 懶紮衣

Movement 1

Sink your hips and turn your torso slightly toward the left front. At the same time, parry the cane up from your front left (southwest) corner to shoulder height. With your eyes following the tip of the cane looking to the front left corner, let your left hand rise (Photo 2-1).

Movement 2

Move the cane in a clockwise curve from the left front, across your centerline, to your right front corner as if you are parrying an incoming weapon targeting your face. At the same time, shift your weight to your left foot and lift your left palm to a ward-off position to your left front (Photo 2-2).

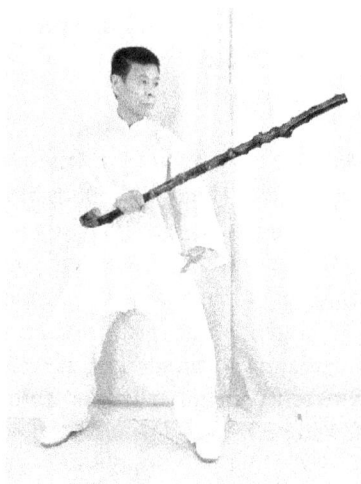

Photo 2-1

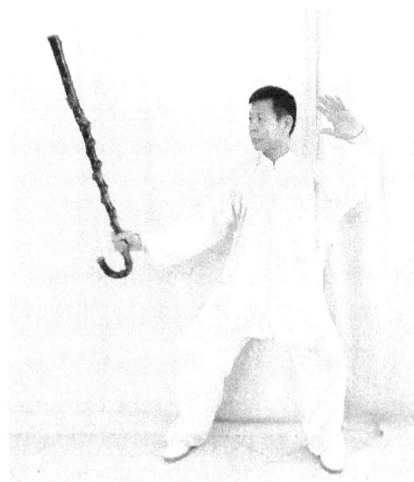

Photo 2-2

Movement 3

Turn your torso to your right and continue to move the cane in a clockwise curve to your right rear corner. Step your right foot to the right side and turn your right palm face up with the cane horizontally guarding your right side (west). At the same time, close your left palm in front of your chest (Photo 2-3).

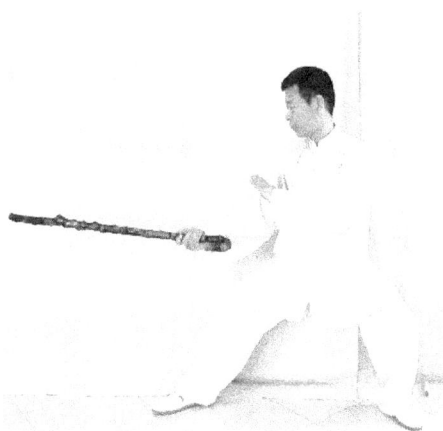

Movement 4

Turn your torso to your left and sweep the cane from the right across your frontline to your left front, and thrust the cane toward your left front. At the same time, rotate your right hand with the knuckles facing up. You are in a horseback riding stance with a little more weight on your left leg (Photo 2-4).

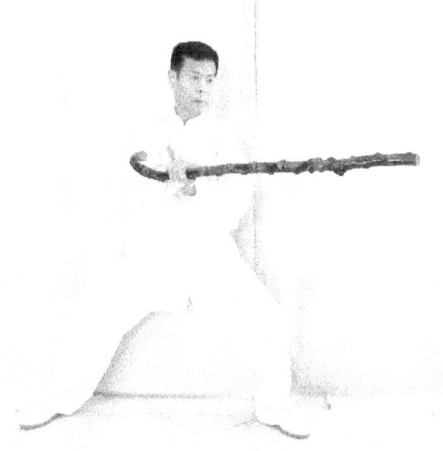

Photo 2-3

Photo 2-4

Movement 5

Move the cane above your head horizontally and pull your right hand from the left front to your right front as you turn your body facing forward. Drop the left hand in front of your belly with the palm facing up and slightly in, and sit in a horseback riding stance (Photo 2-5).

Movement 6

Continue to move the cane to your right front and drop your right hand to waist level. Hold the cane vertically in front of your right knee. At the same time, move your left palm to rest at your left *kua*, the front hip (the juncture of femur and pelvis). Look to your right front (southwest), and maintain a ward-off energy as if the cane were a shield (Photo 2-6).

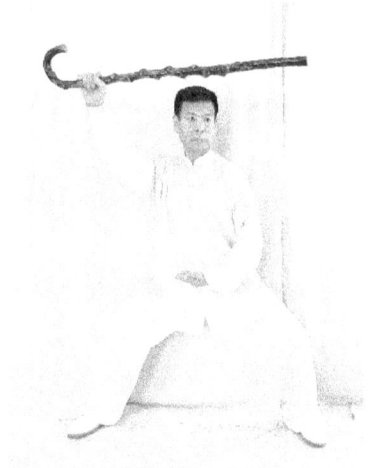

Photo 2-5

Key Points

1) The cane is parried clockwise one-and-a-half circles before settling down in front of your right front corner. With your torso's turning, the circle becomes three-dimensional and extends from your left front to right rear.

2) Use your dantian rotation to drive your torso's turn for the cane circle.

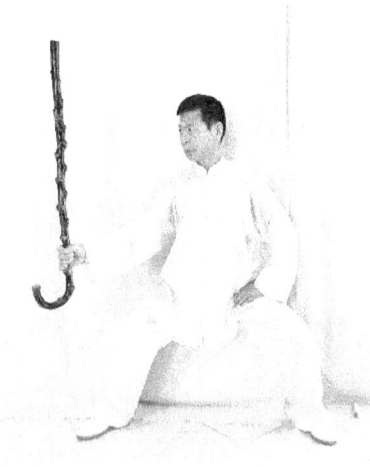

Photo 2-6

Posture 3: Six-Seal & Four-Close 六封四閉

Movement 1

Shift weight to your left foot and deflect the cane tip downward in front of your right leg as if to block out an incoming weapon targeting the right knee. At the same time, move your left palm to guard the front chest (Photo 3-1). Continue to move the cane across your front lower belly to the front of your left shoulder with the tip of the cane spinning up and the left palm pressing on the front of the cane (Photo 3-2).

Movement 2

Shift weight to your right foot and turn your torso toward the right front corner. At the same time, close your left foot a half step and push the tip of the cane (peck) to the right front (southwest). Keep the tip of the cane at face height (Photo 3-3).

Key Points

1) The pecking of the cane tip rides on the clockwise spinning energy and the flow from shifting your body weight.

2) At the end of the pose, maintain the ward-off energy to achieve the meaning of six-sealing and four-closing.

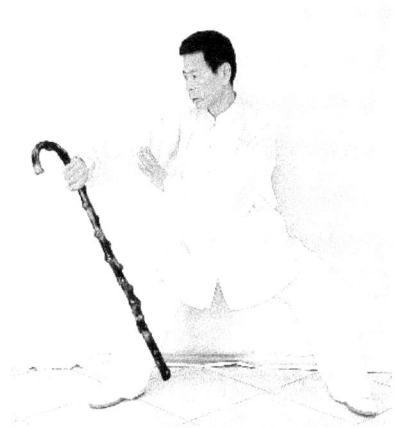

Photo 3-1

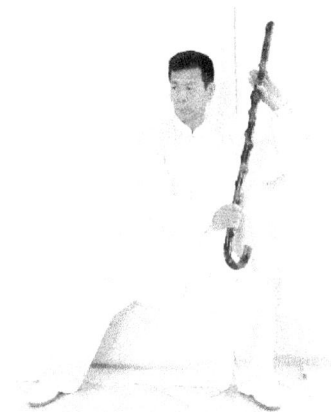

Photo 3-2

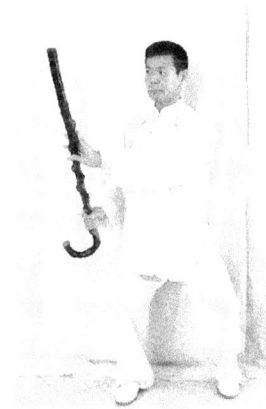

Photo 3-3

Posture 4: Single Whip 單鞭

Movement 1

Turn your torso slightly to the right side and parry the cane tip downward under your right arm to protect your right rib side. Next, turn your torso slightly back to the front right corner to spin the hook of the cane counterclockwise from the side of your right hip to the front of your right shoulder. The cane hook is at head height as you look to your right front corner, the southwest (Photo 4-1).

Movement 2

Make a small counterclockwise circle with the cane hook in front of your right shoulder, then curve it down to outside the right knee as if you are parrying off an incoming weapon targeting your right chest. At the same time, step your left foot to the left and keep your left forearm curved in front of your belly with your left palm facing up. Look to your left front, the southeast (Photo 4-2).

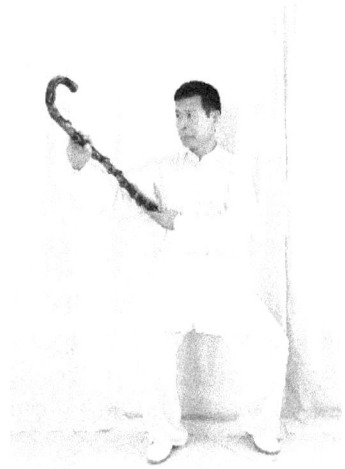

Photo 4-1

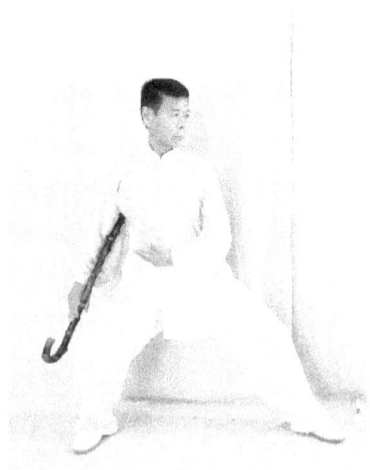

Photo 4-2

Movement 3

Shift weight to your left foot and strike your left elbow to the left. Maintain your right leg and knee in an unlocked position to control the balance (Photo 4-3).

Movement 4

Seeming to pause without really pausing, lift your left palm in front of your chest and sweep it to your left front. At the end of the move, bend your left leg at the knee. Place sixty to seventy percent of your body weight on the left foot, sink your left elbow down, and turn the fingers of your left hand up. Your left palm and chest are facing the left front corner to the southeast (Photo 4-4).

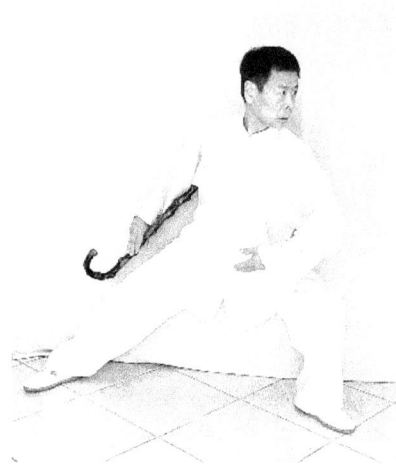

Photo 4-3

Key Points

1) The striking of the hook is powered by your torso's twist and release, rebounding like a spring.

2) At the ending pose, do not stretch your right leg too much. Sink your right hip to keep the right knee unlocked to maintain a rounded crotch for inner energy strength training. This will facilitate your pelvis in a leveled position and give you a comfortable and stable stance.

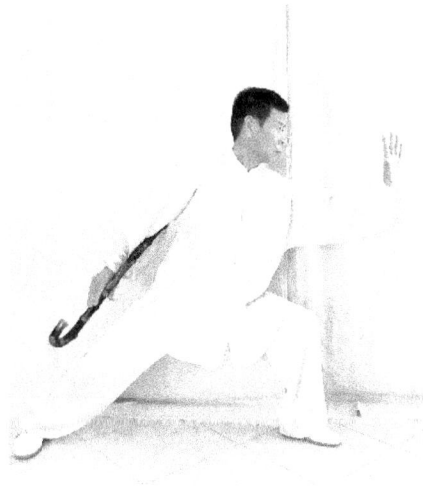

Photo 4-4

Posture 5: Striking Left & Right 左衝右衝

Movement 1

Turn your torso to the left and use your torso to fling the cane from your right back side to the front of your body. The left palm catches the lower part of the cane and the right hand holds the handle end on the top. Keep the cane vertical to guard the front of your body (Photo 5-1).

Movement 2

Twist the cane clockwise into a horizontal position with both palms facing down. Turn your torso facing front (south) in a horseback riding stance with body weight a little more on your right leg. Continue looking to your left side (Photo 5-2).

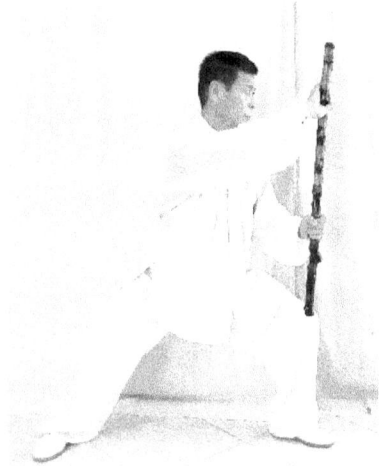

Photo 5-1

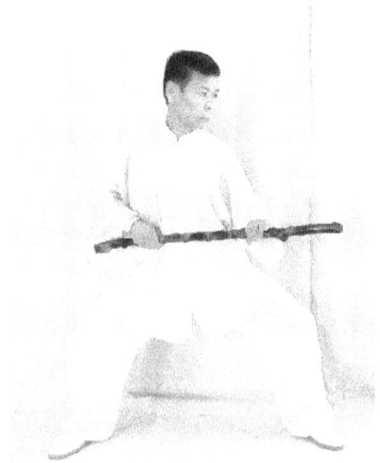

Photo 5-2

Movement 3

Jab the cane tip to your left side (east) and, optionally, you can move your right foot a half step closer. Look in the direction the cane tip is pointing (Photo 5-3).

Movement 4

Step to your right side (west) with your right foot and jab the cane hook end to your right following with a half step with your left foot. Look in the direction the cane hook is striking (Photo 5-4).

Key Points

1) Use your waist-twisting power to bring the cane out from your right back side into a left side block.

2) The half-step flow is important to power the left and right strikes. It is called *gen-bu* 跟步, "following-up steps" in tai chi or martial arts and is used to create an inertial force.

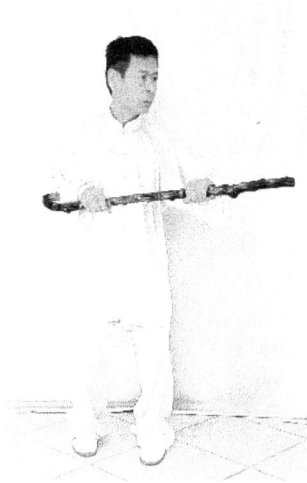

Photo 5-3

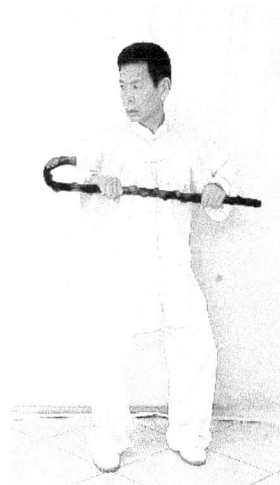

Photo 5-4

Posture 6: Wrapping Head with the Cane 纏頭杖

Movement 1
Raise the cane above your head and turn your torso to the left as if you are fencing up an incoming weapon targeting your face. Hold the cane diagonally in front of your head for protection with the left hand holding the lower end (Photo 6-1).

Movement 2
Turn the cane into a vertical position with the right hand on top and left hand on the bottom. At the same time, turn the torso facing the left (east) and parry the cane to your left side (Photo 6-2).

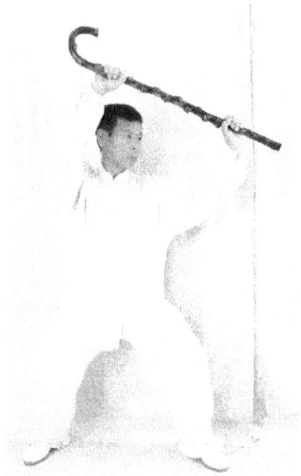
Photo 6-1

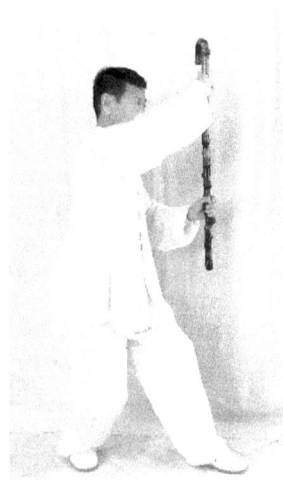
Photo 6-2

Movement 3

Turn your left foot outward pointing to the left rear corner (northeast). At the same time, wrap the cane from the left side behind your back and parry the left palm toward your right rib side. At the end of this pose, your torso and legs are in a spiral position. The right heel is off the floor to assist your torso twist to the left (Photo 6-3).

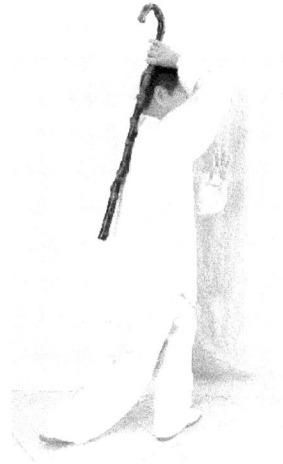

Movement 4

Step to the east with your right foot and bend the knee into a right bow stance (Photo 6-4). At the same time, move your left palm toward the left upper corner above your head and sweep the cane to strike to the east side. Your chest is now facing north (Photo 6-5).

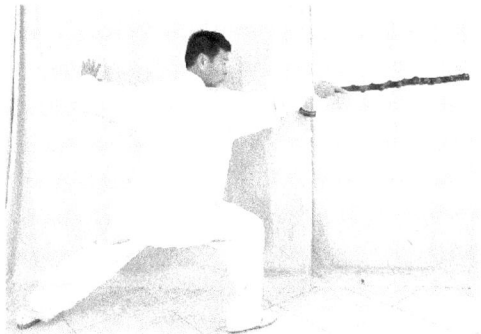

Key Points

1) This is a good example of the tai chi concept in self-defense: defensive move followed by offensive move. Ward off the cane and redirect an incoming weapon before the strike.

2) Use your torso's twist to power the sweeping strike. You can pivot on your left heel to turn out toes or pivot on the ball of the left foot to turn the heel inward.

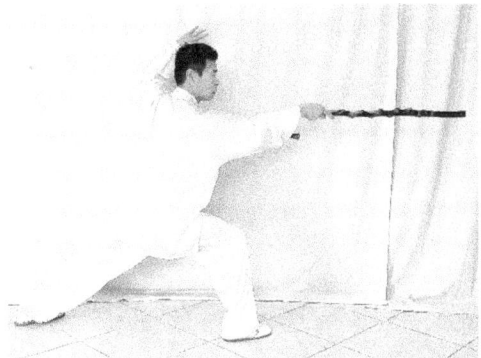

Photo 6-3

Photo 6-4

Photo 6-5

113

Posture 7: Uppercuts Left & Right 護膝杖

Movement 1

Draw back your right foot and rest it momentarily a few inches away from your weighted left foot. At the same time, parry the cane in an upper curve back in front of your chest and close in the left palm around the cane handle to guard the northeast direction (Photo 7-1).

Movement 2

Step your right foot to the east, turn your torso to the right, and lift your left knee. At the same time, move the cane in a counterclockwise circle from your left rear to guard outside your left knee (Photo 7-2). Without stopping, step your left foot to the east and swing the cane to strike forward and upward with the tip of the cane above your head. Bend the left leg at the knee into a bow stance (Photo 7-3).

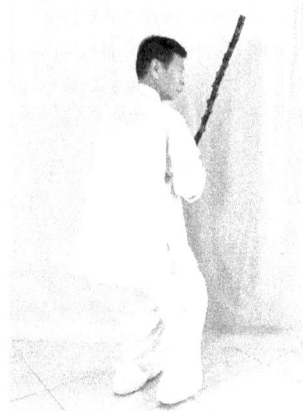

Photo 7-1

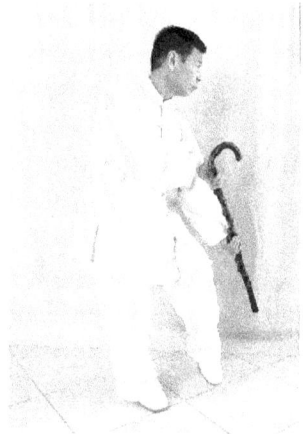

Photo 7-2

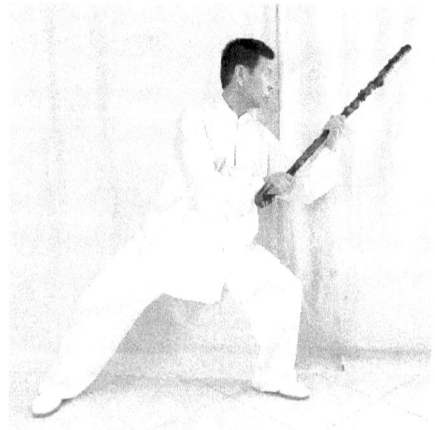

Photo 7-3

Movement 3

Shift weight to your right foot and parry the cane to the front of your right shoulder. Draw back your left foot a half step and rest it momentarily. At the same time, switch your hands with the right hand above your left hand. Look to your left (Photo 7-4).

Movement 4

Step your right foot forward to the east and swing the cane from your right rear in a low curve across and outside your right leg as if to protect your right knee (Photo 7-5). Bend your right leg at the knee into a bow stance and cut the cane forward and upward (Photo 7-6).

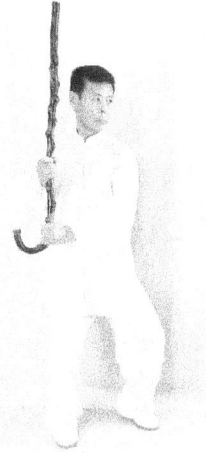

Photo 7-4

Key Points

1) This posture swings the cane around your left and right side in two circles to protect you as you step forward.

2) The cane can also be used for uppercut strikes.

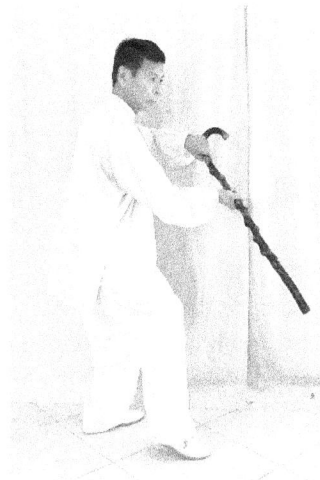

Photo 7-5

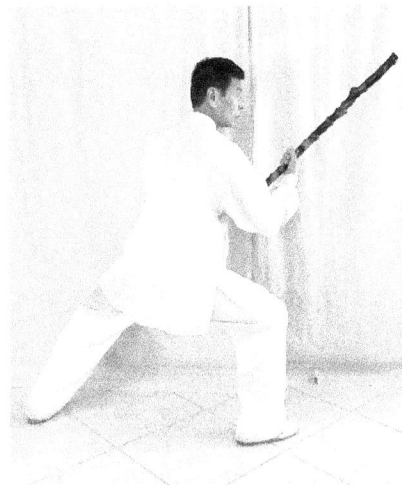

Photo 7-6

Posture 8: Grand Eagle Spreads Wings 雄鷹展翅

Movement 1

Parry the cane to your left, and cross step your left foot behind your right leg. At the same time, hold the cane in front of your chest as if to deflect an incoming weapon targeting your front. Your left hand guards your right rib side under the cover of the hook (Photo 8-1).

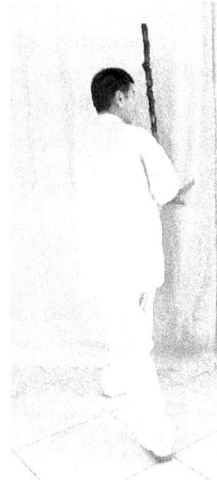

Movement 2

Lean your torso to your left side and strike the cane toward your right lower side. At the same time, push the left palm to your left upper corner. Your body's weight is mainly on your right foot (Photo 8-2).

Key Points

1) Make sure to keep your center of gravity low in the cross stance. Your stance is in a diagonal direction, your left foot is in the southwest direction, and your right foot points northwest.

2) Your left arm and right arm are in a diagonal line. The practice of internal martial arts is based on the balance of opposite movements and flows of intent.

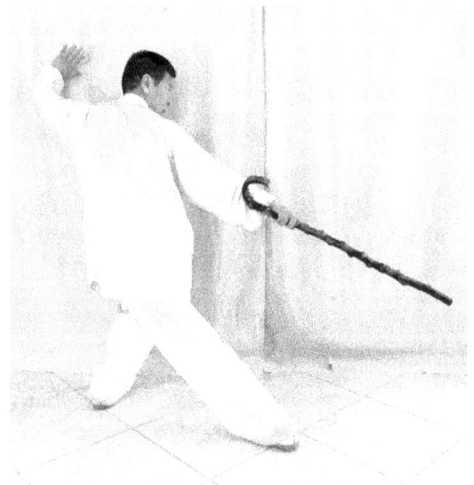

Photo 8-1

Photo 8-2

Posture 9: Embracing the Moon 懷中抱月

Movement 1

Turn your torso to the left and draw your left heel inward by pivoting on the ball of the left foot. Next, ride on the turning flow and turn your right foot inward by pivoting on the right heel to assist your torso to turn 180 degrees. At the same time, sweep the cane from the southeast to the northwest in a low-level circle. Close your left palm in front of your right chest (Photo 9-1).

Movement 2

Continue to sweep the cane across your lower front to your left front. Next, parry the cane up to your left front to guard the southeast direction at head height with your right hand above your head. Round your arm at the elbow and ward off the left palm in front of your left hip, palm facing down. Settle your weight more on the right foot (Photo 9-2).

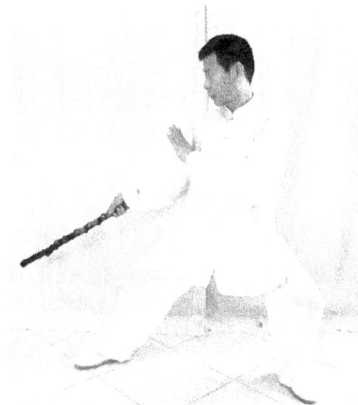

Photo 9-1

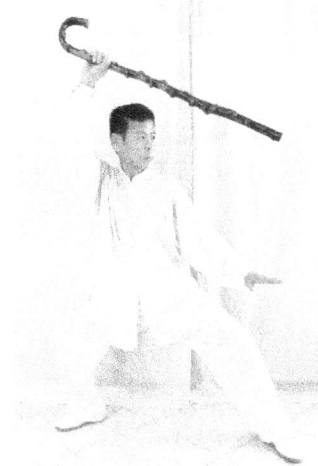

Photo 9-2

Movement 3

Shift the majority of your weight to the left foot as you move the cane from the left front to your right front. At the same time, curve your right hand down and raise your left palm in a clockwise circle as if you are turning a wheel to the right to parry the cane in an upper curve (Photo 9-3).

Movement 4

Drop the right hand toward your left hip to turn the cane diagonally in front of your chest with the tip pointing to the right side. Close the left palm inside the cane handle with the palm facing the handle. Look to the west (Photo 9-4).

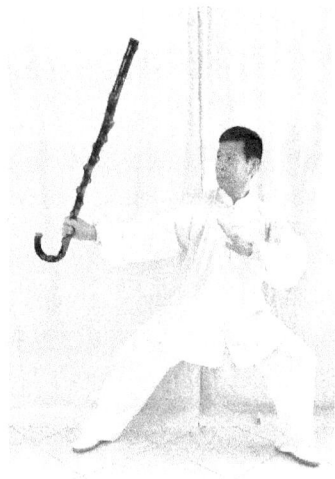

Photo 9-3

Key Points

1) Your arms move from open to close twice in this posture. Alternating open and close to balance the yin and yang is a classic tai chi concept.

2) Keep your arms curved in front of your lower chest while in a horseback riding stance with the left leg weighted a little more.

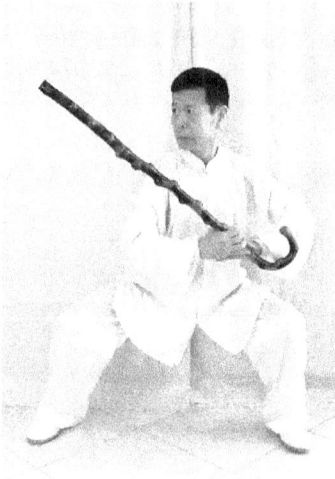

Photo 9-4

Posture 10: Cat Catches Rat 靈貓撲鼠

Movement 1

Parry the cane to the left and turn the cane from pointing to your right to the left in a counterclockwise, downward circle to protect your left knee. At the same time, shift weight to your right leg and move your left foot in with the ball touching the ground a few inches away from the right foot (Photo 10-1).

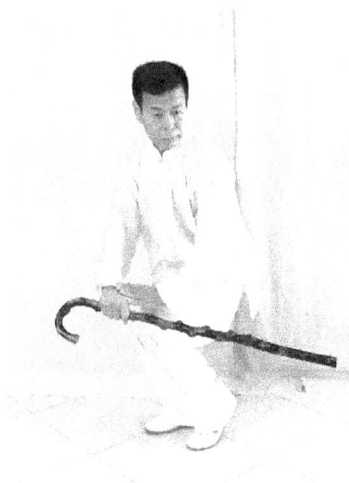

Movement 2

Turn your torso to the right and step your left foot in an inward curve to the northwest direction. Follow your body's direction turning to sweep the cane from your left hip side to the back of your right shoulder. Keep the hook above your head with the tip end lower at shoulder level. Keep the weight on your left foot while twisting the torso. Look back to your right (Photo 10-2).

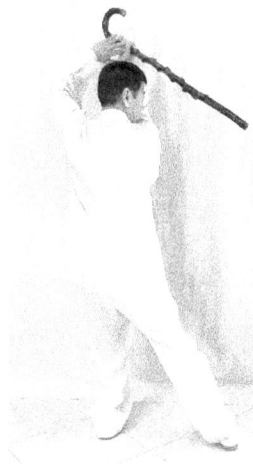

Photo 10-1

Photo 10-2

Movement 3

Pivot on your left heel to curve in the toes of the left foot, and turn your torso right to face the east side. At the same time, lift your right leg and lower both hands to parry the cane down to your right side. Keep the cane guarding outside your right knee (Photo 10-3).

Movement 4

Step your right foot to the east and bend the right knee into a right bow stance. Thrust the cane toward the floor (Photo 10-4).

Key Points

1) The cane swings in a three-dimensional circle following your body's turn from the east side low to the same direction thrusting to the floor.

2) Your right wrist rotates to flip around in Movement 2.

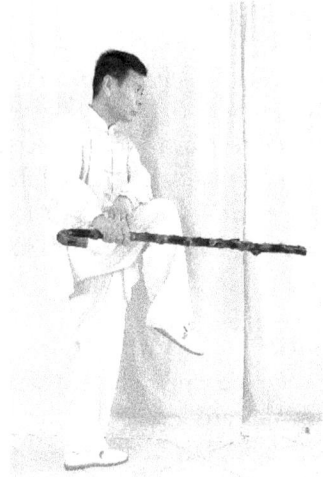

Photo 10-3

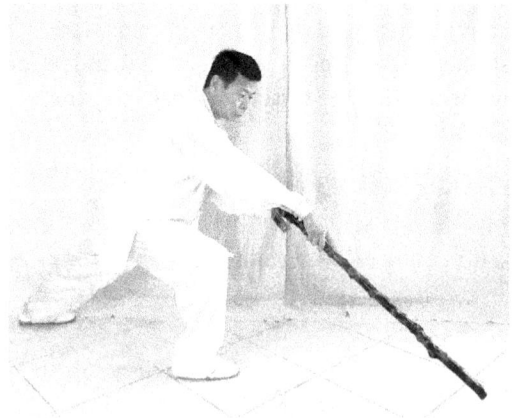

Photo 10-4

Posture 11: Golden Rooster Standing on One Foot 金鷄獨立

Movement 1

Pivot on the right heel and turn the right toes toward the southeast. At the same time, parry the cane upward in a clockwise curve to protect the front of your chest. The cane swings above your head with the tip a little lower (Photo 11-1).

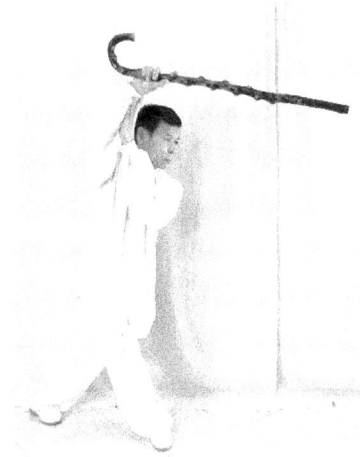

Movement 2

Step your left foot to the front right corner (southeast), and circle the cane down to chest height (Photo 11-2). Seeming to pause without really pausing, lift your right foot into a left rooster stance. Thrust the cane to the east at shoulder height (Photo 11-3).

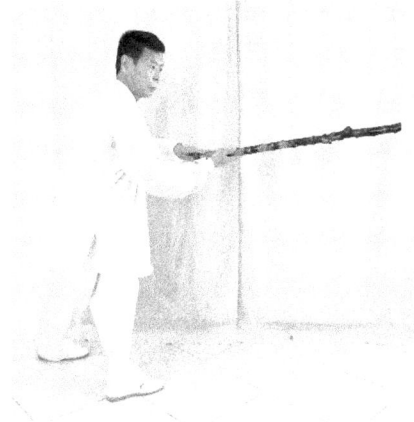

Key Points

1) The left step has to be curved to the right side to avoid the centerline.

2) The cane moves in a small, clockwise circle before thrusting out.

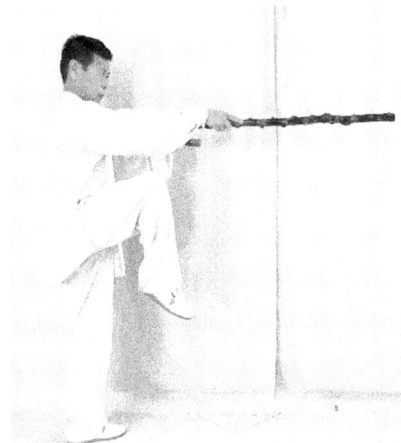

Photo 11-1

Photo 11-2

Photo 11-3

Posture 12: Whipping Sleeves & Slamming Cane 翻花舞袖

Movement 1
Hop forward on your left foot and extend your right leg in front of you. At the same time, lift the tip of the cane back above your head (Photo 12-1). The cane seems to pause without really pausing. Chop the cane to the east at shoulder height as your right foot steps down, and bend the right knee into a right bow stance (Photo 12-2).

Movement 2
Parry the cane up in a clockwise half circle on your right side and then press the cane down guarding the outside of your hip. At the same time, shift your weight into a horseback riding stance. Ward off with your left palm in front of your belly, and look to the east side (Photo 12-3).

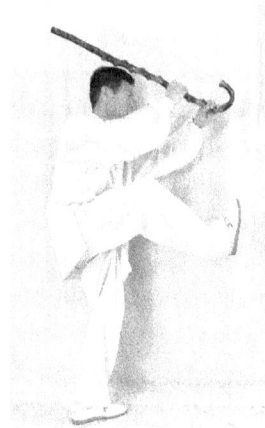

Photo 12-1

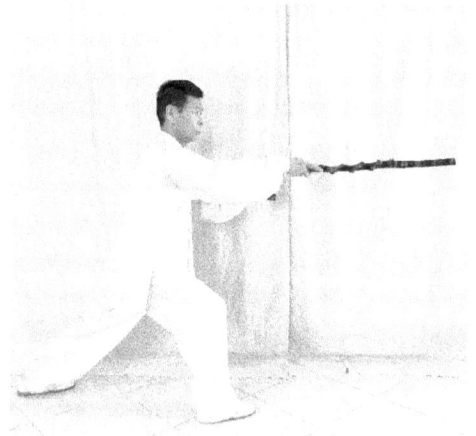

Photo 12-2

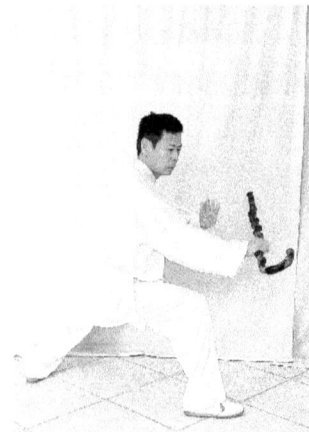

Photo 12-3

Movement 3

Turn your torso to the left and ward off with the left arm to protect your left side at head height. Lift your left knee to start the turning-around jump while the right hand holds the cane still at the right lower side (Photo 12-4).

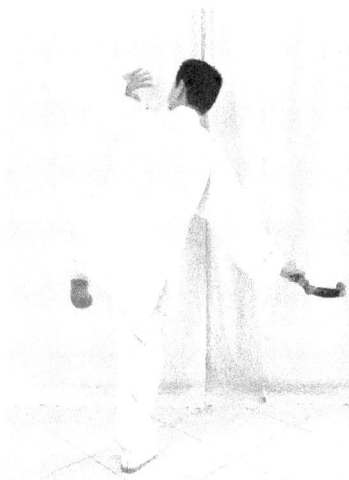

Movement 4

Continue turning to your left side and jump up with the right foot, letting your body turn 360 degrees in the air, and land in a horseback riding stance. At the same time, like a spinning wheel, swing the cane high with your torso's spinning and then strike it down horizontally to the outside of your right knee. Your left palm circles from high to low and then high again in front of the left side of your head (Photo 12-5).

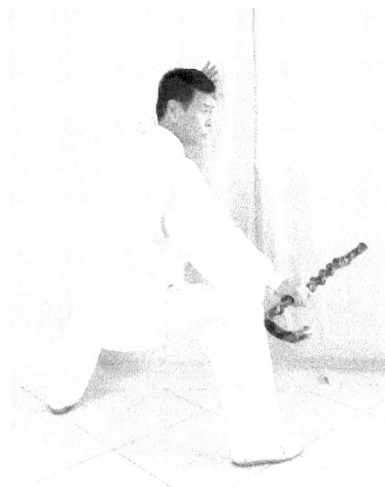

Photo 12-4

Key Points

1) This 360-degree turn and jump can be a forward (to the east) jump for offensive strike or a backward jump for defensive block to move away from an aggressive attacker.

2) Optionally, if you are uncomfortable making the jump turn, just turn to the left and step with the right foot, then the left foot, then the right foot again to turn a whole circle.

Photo 12-5

Posture 13: Overturn the Ocean 海底翻花

Movement 1

Shift weight to the left foot and draw your right foot back. At the same time, parry the cane vertically with the hook above your head across your front centerline to your left shoulder. The left palm moves down and parries to your right rib side (Photo 13-1).

Movement 2

Lift your right knee and strike the cane down horizontally to the outside of your right leg. At the same time, move your left hand from a lower curve across your belly and up to the left side of your head. Look down at your right side (Photo 13-2).

Key Points

1) This is a rooster stance with the left foot on the floor. Make sure to lower your body weight onto your left foot before lifting up the right knee.

2) Striking the cane down with your right hand has to be balanced with the opposite upward movement of your left fist.

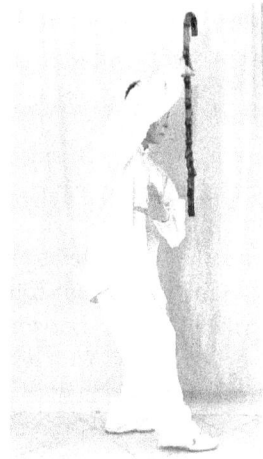

Photo 13-1

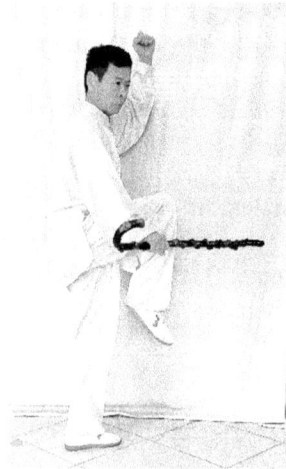

Photo 13-2

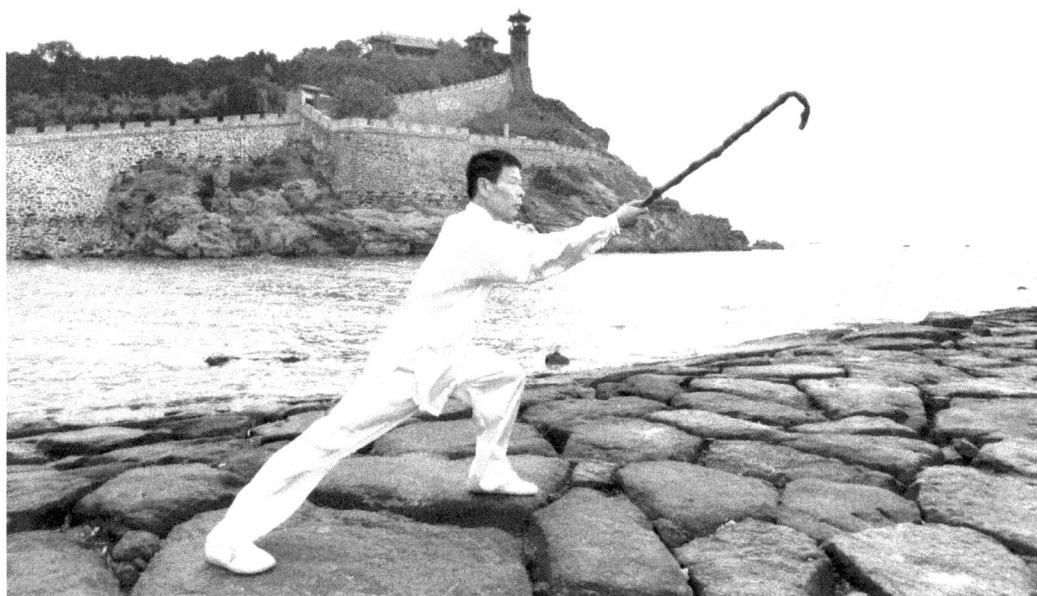

橫掃千軍

Batting a Home Run

Posture 14: Dragon's Tail Stirring Water 黃龍三攬水

Movement 1

Step to the east with your right foot and follow with a half step with your left foot. At the same time, parry the cane up horizontally in front of your body at shoulder height. Slide your right hand toward the hook and drop your left hand with the palm resting on your left waist area. Look to the east side (Photo14-1).

Movement 2

Step back to the west with your left foot while parrying the cane to the east with the tip of the cane pointing to the northeast corner (Photo 14-2). Seeming to pause without really pausing, rotate the cane tip in front of your body in a clockwise circle from your top left front corner to the lower left front corner. At the same time, shift weight to your left foot and step the right foot back behind your left leg into a crossing stance (Photo 14-3).

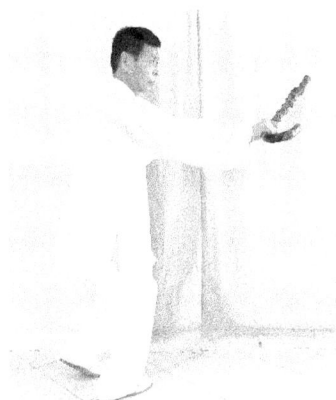

Photo 14-1

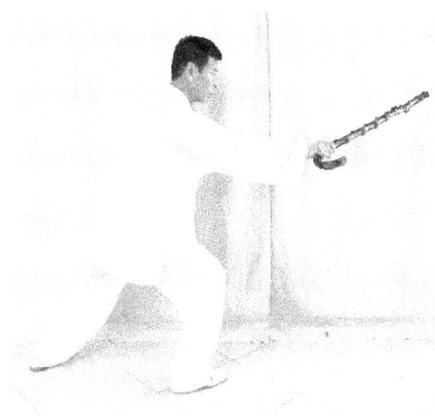

Photo 14-2

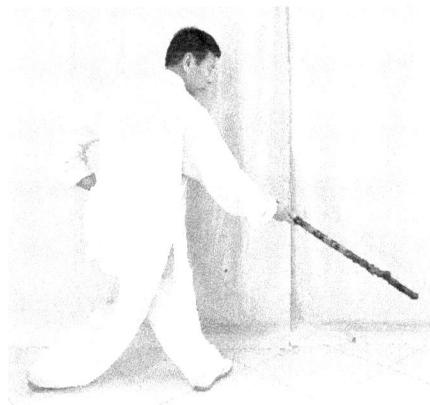

Photo 14-3

Movement 3

Repeat Movement 2 two more times. Your left palm is on your left waist area at all times. Eyes follow the cane circle around looking to the east side (Photos 14-4 to 14-7).

Key Points

1) This is a posture to deflect an aggressive attacker by stepping backward with the cane covering your front. Imagine that you are parrying high and low in a linked coiling motion as if a dragon's tail were stirring water.

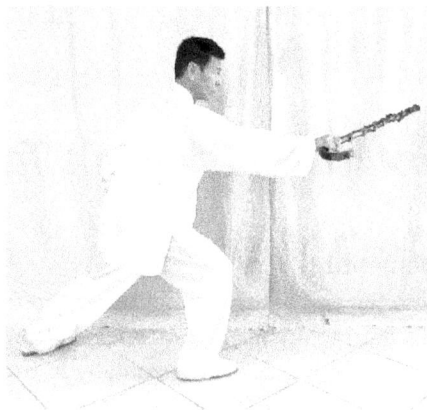

Photo 14-4

2) The crossing stance creates a downward-pressing, spiral energy rooted in the feet to power the cane circles.

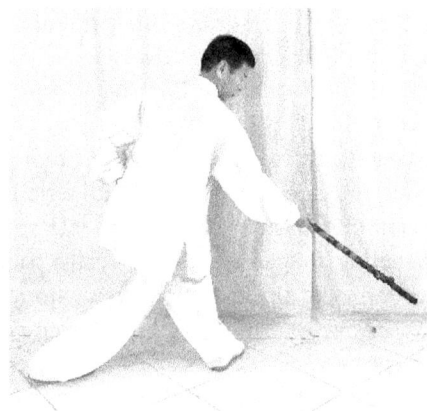

Photo 14-5

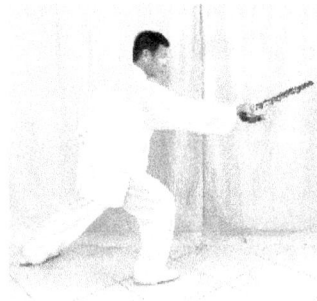

Photo 14-6

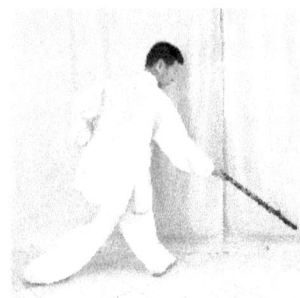

Photo 14-7

Posture 15: Pinwheel Cane 雙舞花

Movement 1

Shift weight to your right leg, turn your torso to the right, and turn your right heel inward by pivoting on the right toes. Next, turn your left toes inward by pivoting on the left heel. At the same time, spin the cane tail up from your lower left side with your left hand held at the middle of the cane (northeast) and ending at the front of your left shoulder (Photo 15-1).

Movement 2

Continue to turn your torso to the right toward the southwest, and shift weight to your left foot with your right heel up in an empty stance. Slide your right hand up close to the left hand around the middle of the cane, and parry the cane tail across your chest center to the outside of your right shoulder (Photo 15-2).

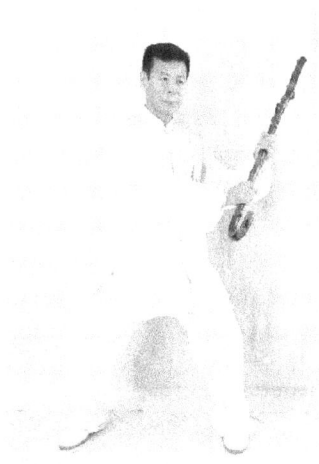

Photo 15-1

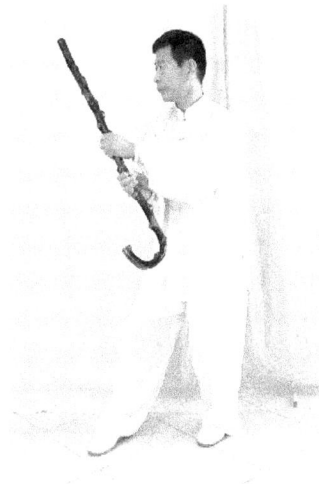

Photo 15-2

Movement 3

Rotate your right wrist to spin the cane tail down to the outside of your right hip and the cane hook up in front of your chest, eyes following the cane's tail (Photo 15-3). Without stopping, rotate your right wrist to spin the cane tail up from your right hip side in an upper curve across your front to your left hip side (Photo 15-4). Then repeat the same pinwheel circle a few more times.

Key Points

1) Pinwheel the cane by your torso's turning and wrist rotation to make smooth circles. Spin the cane with a figure-eight loop at least three to four times in the southwest direction. Imagine you are using the cane pinwheel to deflect away incoming weapons.

2) Make sure your hands hold the middle part of the cane for weight balance for spinning.

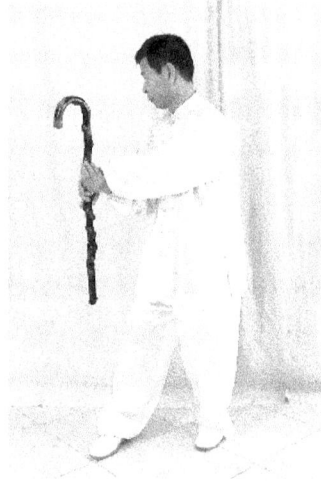

Photo 15-3

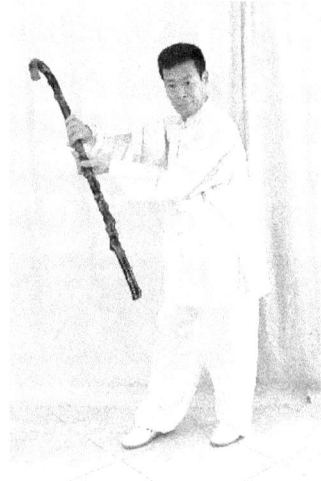

Photo 15-4

Posture 16: Fair Lady Works at Shuttles 玉女穿梭

Movement 1

At the end of the pinwheel, stomp your right foot and immediately lift your left foot. At the same time, parry the cane to guard the outside of your right hip with the tail of the cane pointing to the southwest (Photo 16-1).

Movement 2

Step your left foot to the southwest corner and bend the left knee into a left bow stance. At the same time, parry your left arm up in front of your head, rotate the left palm facing forward, and then thrust the cane to the southwest corner with your right hand rotating your palm to face up. The cane is horizontal at the heart level (Photo 16-2).

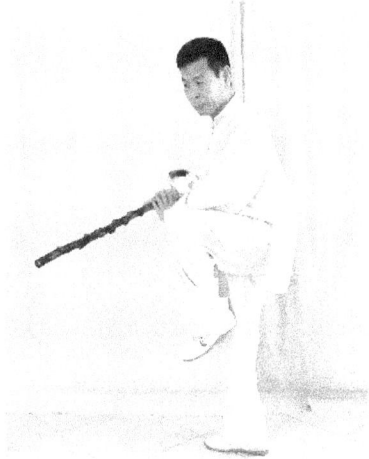

Photo 16-1

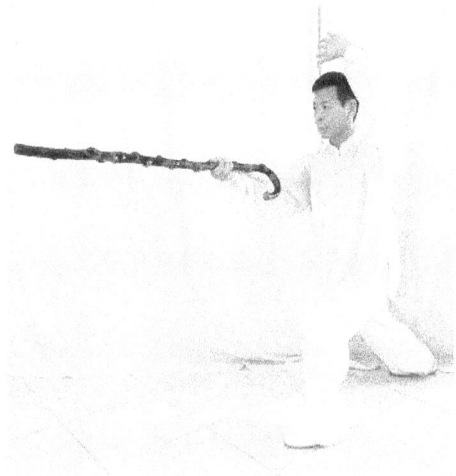

Photo 16-2

Movement 3

Shift your weight to the middle of your feet, turn the toes of the left foot inward forty-five degrees, and squat into a horseback riding stance. At the same time, flip the cane with your right palm facing down, move the left palm back pressing to the middle of the cane, and hold the cane in front of your chest horizontally (Photo 16-3).

Movement 4

Continue to turn your torso to the right and turn your left toes inward as much as you can, about 180 degrees from the northwest to southeast. Step your right foot to the southeast corner with the cane guarding in front of your right leg, still keeping your left palm in front of your chest (Photo 16-4). Without a stop, parry the cane up and hold it horizontally above your head. At the same time, push your left palm out to the southeast corner (Photo 16-5).

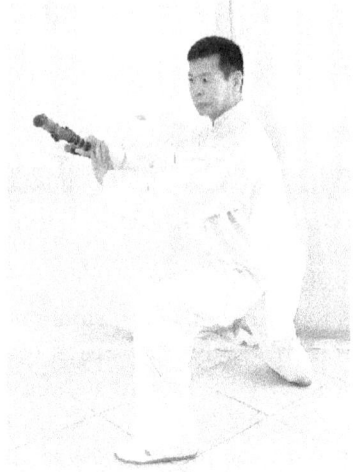

Photo 16-3

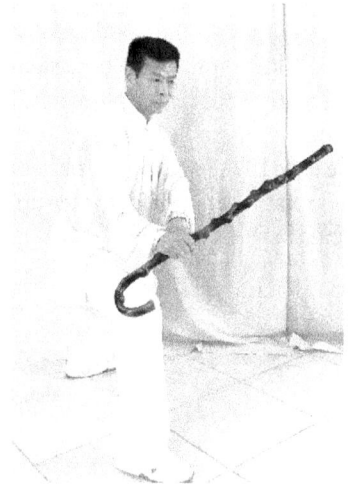

Photo 16-4

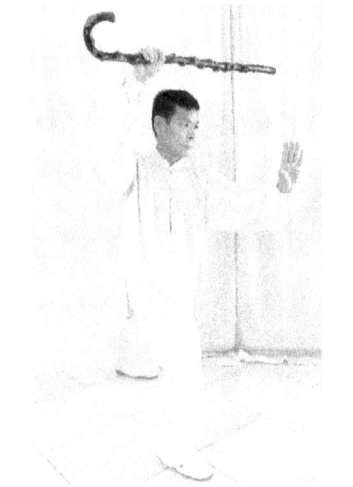

Photo 16-5

Movement 5

Shift weight back to your left foot and draw your right foot halfway back with the ball of the right foot touching the floor in a right empty stance. At the same time, turn your torso to the left and paddle the cane tail down to the front of your left hip (Photo 16-6).

Movement 6

Spin up the cane tail in a clockwise circle to the front of your right shoulder (Photo 16-7). Without a stop, turn your torso to the right and continue to spin the cane tail down to the outside of your right hip. Spin the cane with a figure-eight loop in the southeast corner. Optionally, you can spin the figure-eight loop a few more times (Photo 16-8).

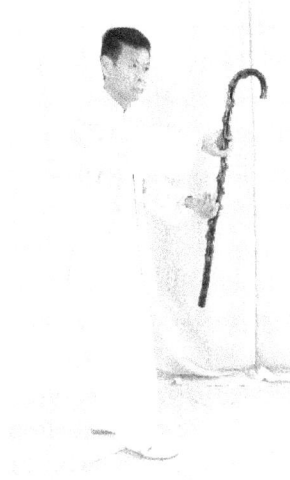

Photo 16-6

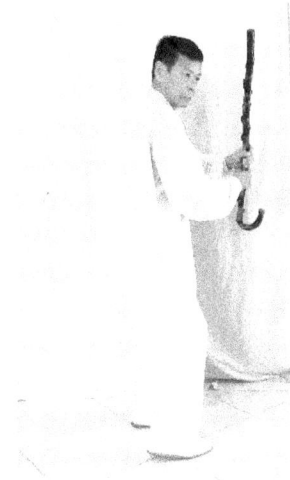

Photo 16-7

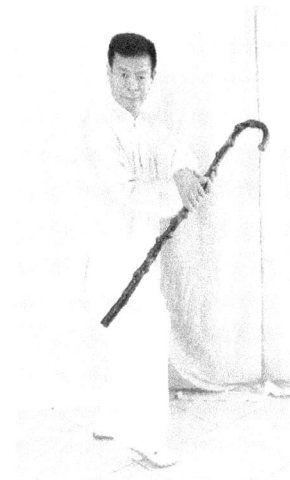

Photo 16-8

Movement 7

At the end of the pinwheel, when the cane tail is low in front of your left hip (Photo16-9), stomp your right foot and immediately lift your left foot. At the same time, parry the cane to guard the outside of your right hip with the tail of the cane pointing to the northeast (Photo 16-10).

Movement 8

Step to the northeast corner with your left foot, and bend the left knee into a left bow stance. At the same time, parry your left arm up in front of your head and rotate your left palm facing forward. Thrust the cane to the northeast corner. The cane is horizontal at the heart level (Photo 16-11).

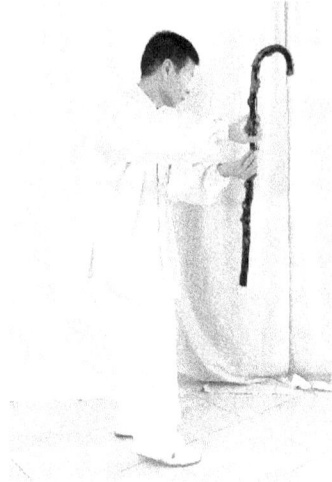

Photo 16-9

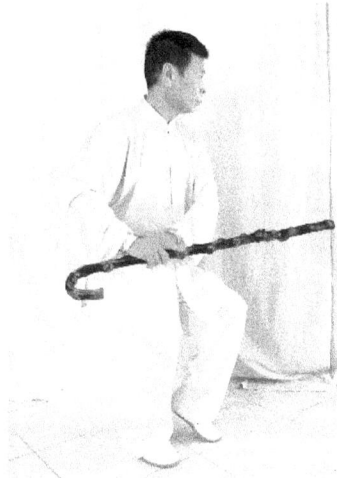

Photo 16-10

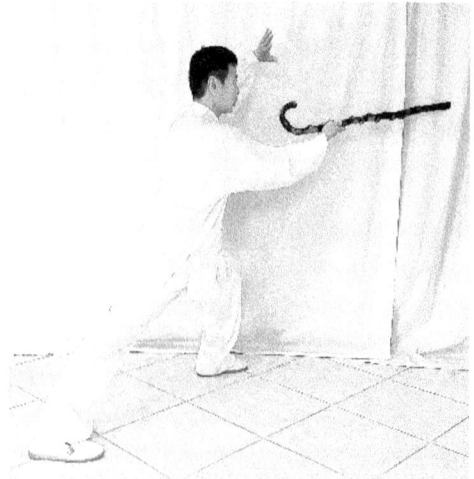

Photo 16-11

Movement 9

Movement 9 is a repeat of Movement 3 and Movement 4, with different directions.

Shift your weight to the middle of your feet and turn the left toes inward forty-five degrees, and squat into a horseback riding stance. At the same time, flip the cane with your right palm facing down, left palm moving back, and press the palm to the middle part of the cane. Hold the cane in front of your chest horizontally (Photo 16-12). Continue to turn your torso to the right and turn your left toes inward as much as you can, about 180 degrees from the southeast to northwest. Step to the northwest corner with your right foot with the cane guarding in front of your right leg. Continue to keep your left palm in front of your chest (Photo 16-13). Without a stop, parry the cane up and hold it horizontally above your head. At the same time, push out your left palm to the northwest corner (Photo 16-14).

Key Points

1) Alternately, thrust the cane to the southwest and northeast corners, and push your left palm to the southeast and northwest corners.

2) Make sure to adjust your feet to facilitate your body turning around, and use your torso's turn to spin the cane looping around.

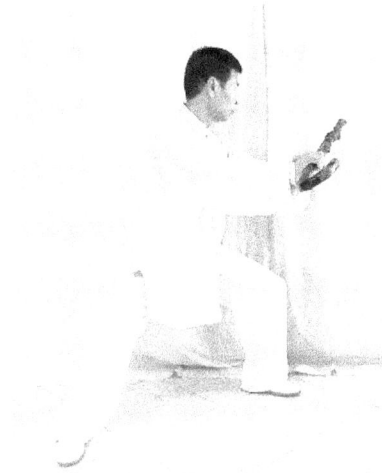

Photo 16-12

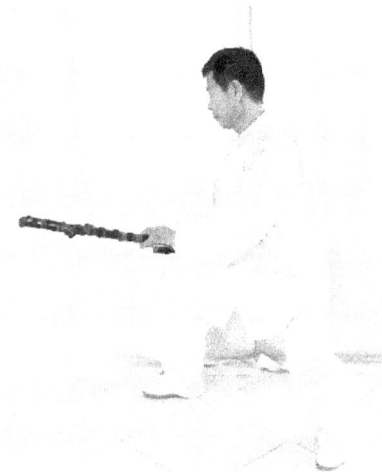

Photo 16-13

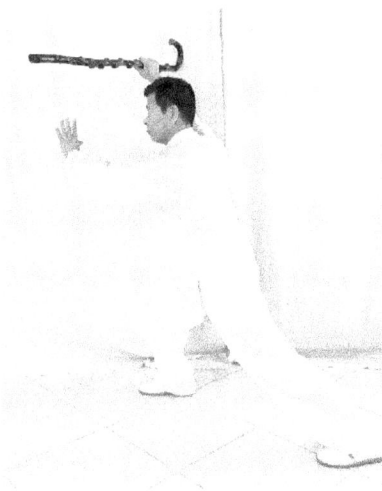

Photo 16-14

Posture 17: Batting a Home Run 橫掃千軍

Movement 1

Bring your left hand to hold the cane tail down toward your chest and shift weight to your left foot. Turn your torso to the left to parry the cane hook in front of your head for an outward curve from the northwest corner toward your left (Photo 17-1).

Movement 2

Shift weight to your right leg and continue the circle of the cane hook from your left front to the back of your head to parry to the right rear corner (Photo 17-2). Without a stop, slide your right hand to the tail of the cane and extend the cane hook to the right rear lower corner (northwest). At the same time, extend your left palm to the opposite southeast corner to balance the hook. You are in a right bow stance (Photo 17-3).

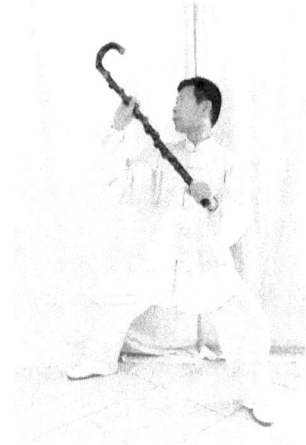

Photo 17-1

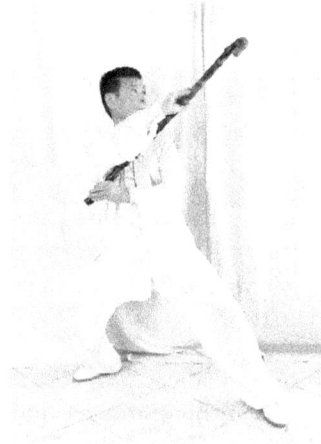

Photo 17-2

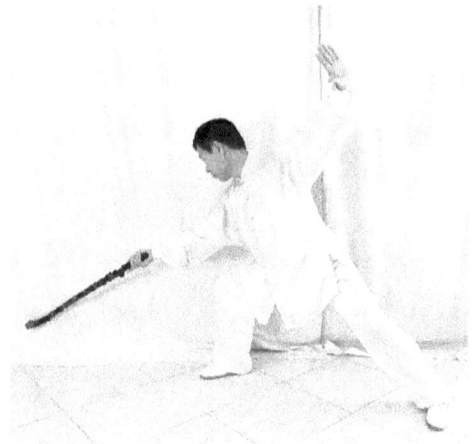

Photo 17-3

Movement 3

Shift weight back to your left leg, pull your right hand back to the front of your left shoulder to hook the cane handle diagonally upward using the cane handle to hook an opponent's leg up and pull him off balance (Photo 17-4).

Movement 4

Swing the cane clockwise a half circle above your head as if you are deflecting away an incoming weapon targeting your head. Hold the cane in front to guard your forehead. At the same time, pull up your right foot and stomp a few inches behind your left foot. Immediately lift your left heel into an empty stance. Look at the southeast corner (Photo 17-5).

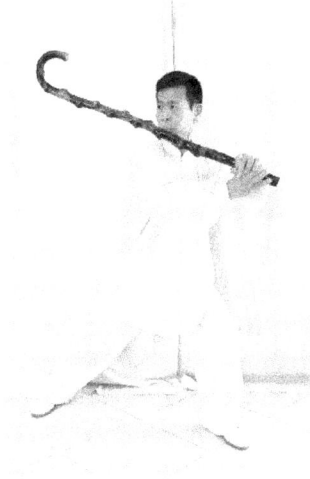

Photo 17-4

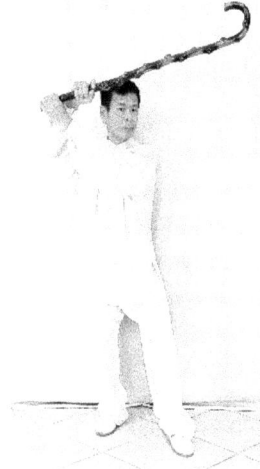

Photo 17-5

Movement 5

Step to the east with your left foot and continue swinging the cane clockwise from the front of your head to your right rear corner as if you are swinging a baseball bat with the cane in front of your right shoulder (Photo 17-6).

Movement 6

Seeming to pause without actually pausing, shift weight to your left foot, bend the left leg into a left bow stance, and whack the cane handle to the front southeast corner with the hook higher than your head. The cane is diagonally in front of your torso lined up with the extended right leg (Photo 17-7).

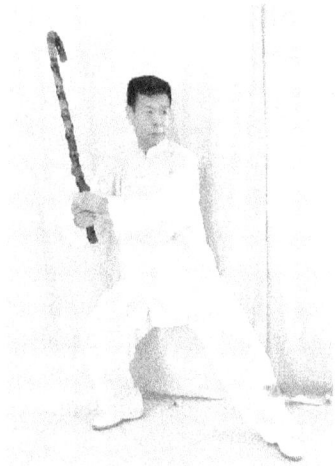

Photo 17-6

Key Points

1) This posture delivers a heavy blow to your front upper area with your body's forward momentum to the strike.

2) Optionally, you can use a shuffle step by dragging your right foot; also, you can hop forward with your left foot to move closer so the strike reaches the target.

3) The cane moves in a large three-dimensional circle following your torso's turning on your right side.

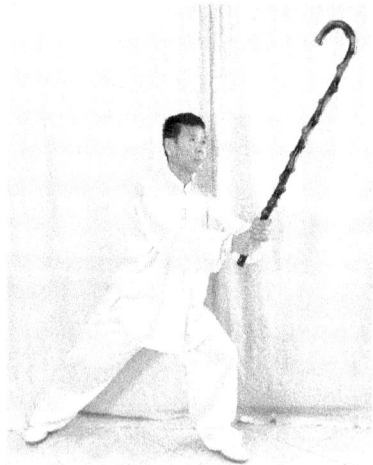

Photo 17-7

Posture 18: Ruthless Lord Holds Up Flag 霸王舉旗

Movement 1

Hold the cane vertically in front of your left shoulder with the left hand at the bottom. With the cane hook on top, lift your right foot and stand on your left foot, looking to the right, the west (Photo 18-1).

Movement 2

Step your right foot to the west and circle the cane hook down to your left side. As the hook lowers to your calf level, lift your left foot as if you were parrying away an incoming weapon targeting your left knee. Pay attention that your arms are crossing at this moment with your right hand low (Photo 18-2). Immediately turn your torso to the right and step to the west with your left foot. Continue to turn your torso to face the east side with the cane following your body and swinging up to guard in front of your chest (Photo 18-3).

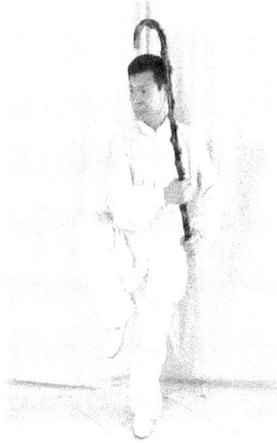

Photo 18-1

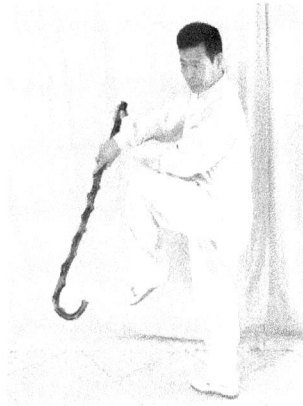

Photo 18-2

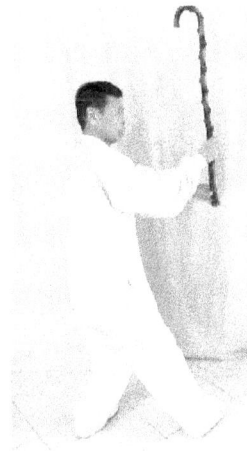

Photo 18-3

Movement 3

Deflect the cane down from the front toward your right side and step back with your right foot to the west, as if you were using the cane to protect your right leg. Shift weight to your right foot with the cane low at the outside of your right leg (Photo 18-4).

Movement 4

Circle the cane up from the back of your right side and lift your left heel as if you were holding a flagstaff (Photo 18-5).

Key Points

1) Optionally, you can jump and turn to the right on your left foot. It can be a long distance leap or a small circle spin depending on the situation.

2) At the end of the posture, the cane is held in front of your chest with a ward-off energy ready for reaction.

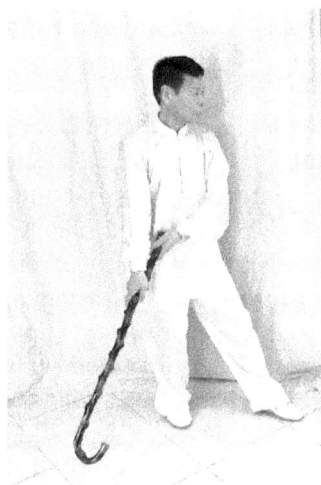

Photo 18-4

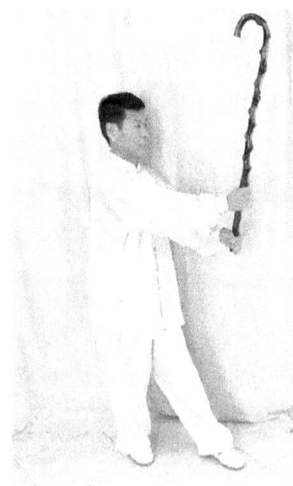

Photo 18-5

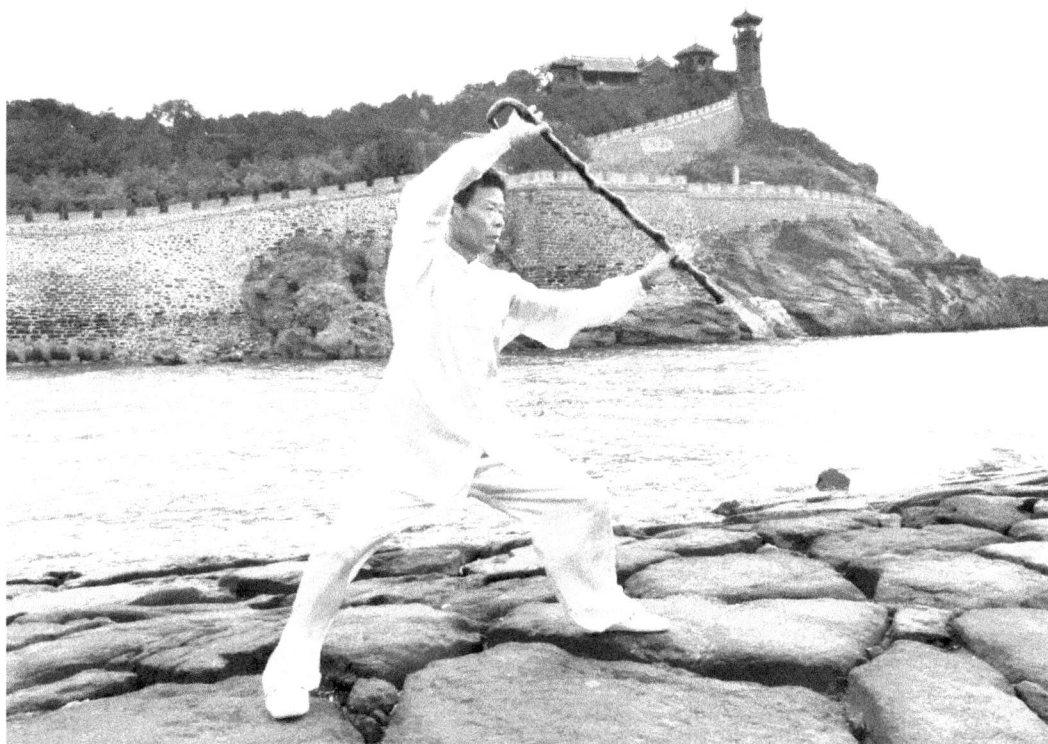

青龍入海

Dragon Descends into Ocean

Section III

Posture 19: Strike Low & Strike High 震腳雙砸

Movement 1

Turn your left foot outward to the northeast corner and deflect the cane handle downward to your left front with your torso turning to the left. Your legs are crossed. You may lift the right heel to smooth the torso's left twist (Photo 19-1).

Movement 2

Swing the cane up in a large clockwise circle from your back left corner (northwest) across your front upper corner to your lower right front. At the same time, turn your torso to the right and step your right foot to the east with the right toes pointing to the right front corner (southwest). Cross your legs and twist your torso to the right with the left heel off the floor (Photo 19-2).

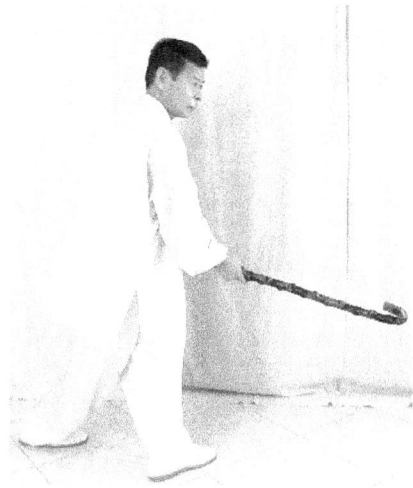
Photo 19-1

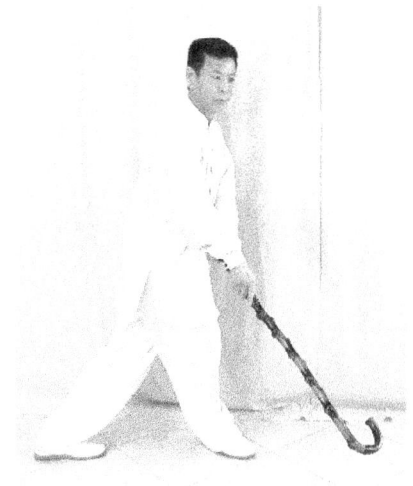
Photo 19-2

Movement 3

Turn your body to the right and step your left foot to the east. At the same time, swing the cane up in a counterclockwise half circle from your right side (west), and hold the cane in front of your right shoulder (Photo 19-3). Seeming to pause without really pausing, shift weight forward and bend your left leg at the knee into a lower left bow stance. Whack the cane hook low in front to the southeast corner (Photo 19-4).

Movement 4

Step your right foot just a few inches behind the left foot, then shift weight to the right foot and lift the left heel off the floor. At the same time, deflect the cane from the front southeast across your right side to your right rear corner (northwest). Look to your left (Photo 19-5).

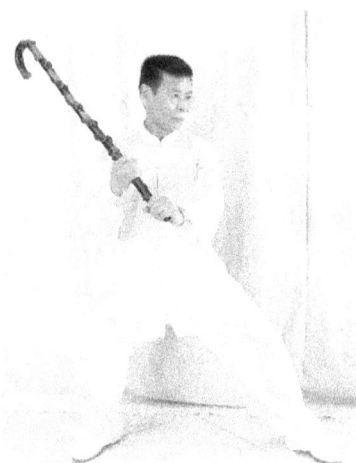

Photo 19-3

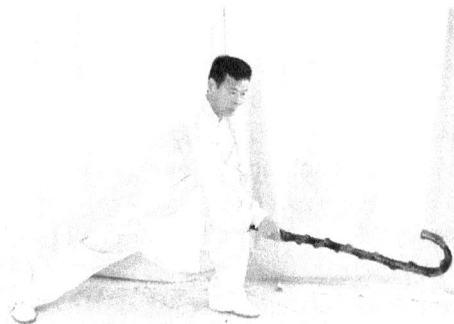

Photo 19-4

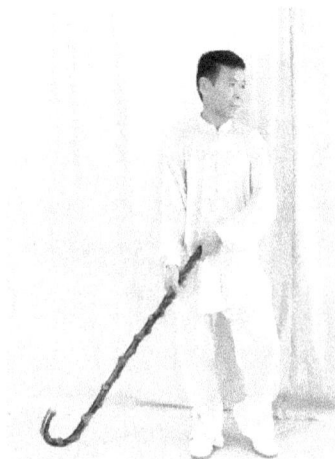

Photo 19-5

Movement 5

Step to the east with your left foot, and at the same time swing the cane up in a counterclockwise half circle from your right side (west). Hold the cane above your right shoulder (Photo 19-6). Seeming to pause without really pausing, shift weight forward and bend your left knee into a left bow stance. Whack the cane hook to your front upper corner toward the southeast (Photo 19-7).

Key Points

1) In these two striking moves, optionally you can move the right foot across your left leg if you need to advance the distance to catch your opponent, or hop or shuffle your right foot to the east side to speed up your action.

2) Use the cane swing momentum and your shifting body weight to power these two strong strikes.

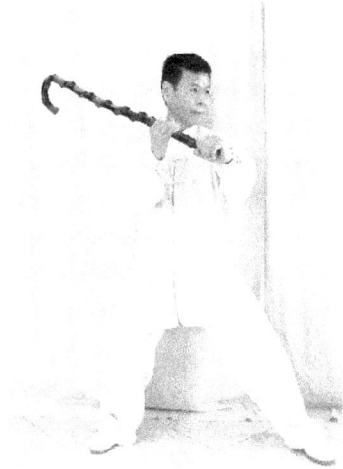

Photo 19-6

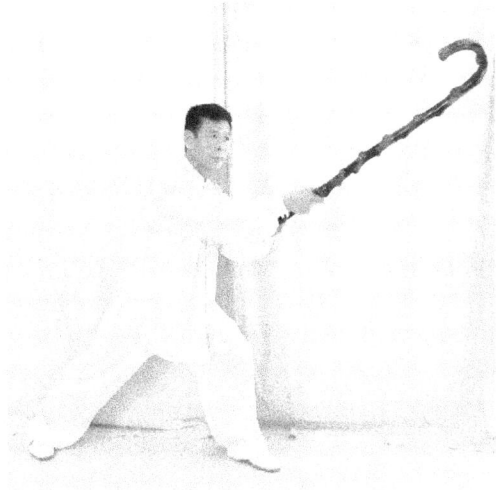

Photo 19-7

Posture 20: Dragon Descends into Ocean 青龍入海

Movement 1
Change your right-hand grip to the area about six inches away from the hook with the palm facing out. At the same time, shift weight slightly to the middle of your feet, and turn the cane diagonally to guard in front of your head with the hook to the southwest and the tail to the northeast (Photo 20-1).

Movement 2
Slide down your left hand eight to ten inches away from the tip of the cane and spin the cane clockwise in front of your head to deflect an incoming weapon to your right side. At the same time, lower your right hand in front of your right chest with the tip of the cane pointing to the southeast corner (Photo 20-2). Seeming to pause without really pausing, shift weight to your right foot and squat as low as you can into a low stance (Photo 20-3).

Key Points
1) Imagine you parry the cane in front of your head and redirect an incoming weapon to the right.

2) Press the cane down to seal it.

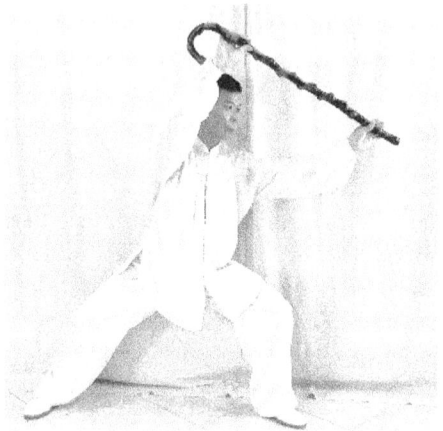

Photo 20-1

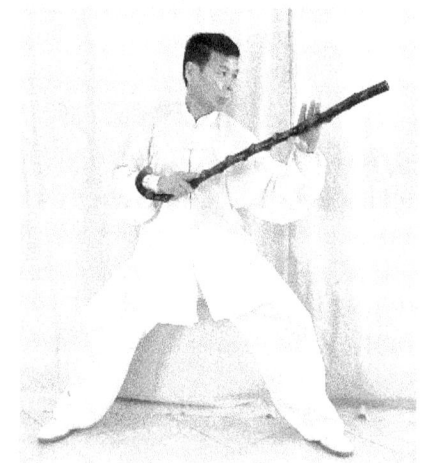

Photo 20-2

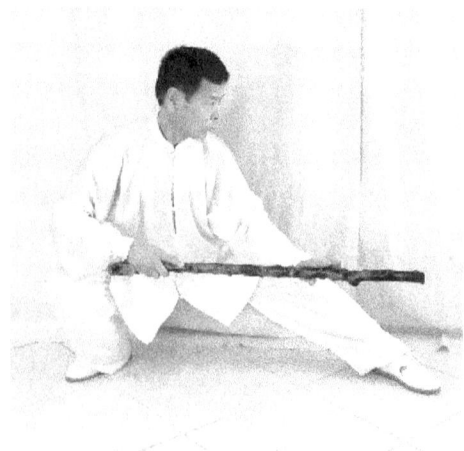

Photo 20-3

Posture 21: Dragon Emerges from Water 青龍出水

Movement 1

Stand up from the low stance with the cane guarding in front of your chest and the tip pointing to the east. Keep your back upright and press down with your waist to create a rebounding energy to help you get up (Photo 21-1).

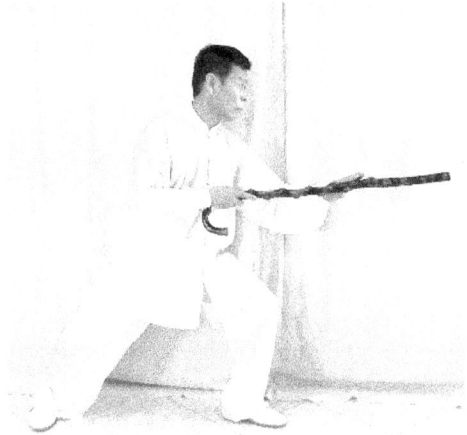

Movement 2

Step your right foot forward but still keep your center of gravity on the back of your left foot. At the same time, extend your right arm and strike the cane to the east with the left palm sliding back along the cane to the cane hook. Your right foot is only a half step in front with the right heel off the floor (Photo 21-2).

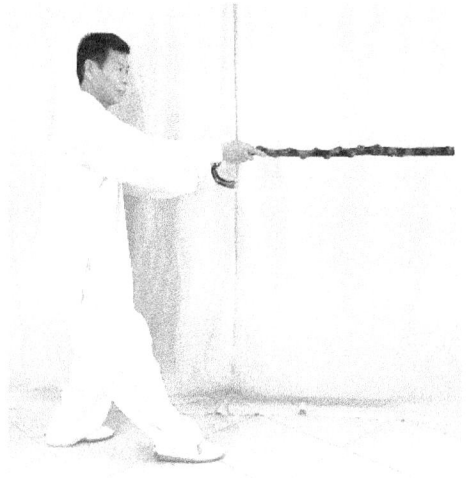

Photo 21-1

Key Points

1) Keep your torso vertical and the cane lined up straight with your right arm in the forward striking pose.

2) Press your left foot on the floor to balance the cane thrusting forward. It is a principle in tai chi that energy is rooted in the feet.

Photo 21-2

Posture 22: Parry Left & Right 迎鋒滾閉

Movement 1

Step back with your right foot and shift weight. At the same time, bend your right wrist and peck the tip of the cane downward. Next, immediately twist the cane in a clockwise half circle in front of you. Hold the cane vertically in front of your chest with the left palm braced at the middle of the cane. Your left heel is off the floor in a left empty stance (Photo 22-1).

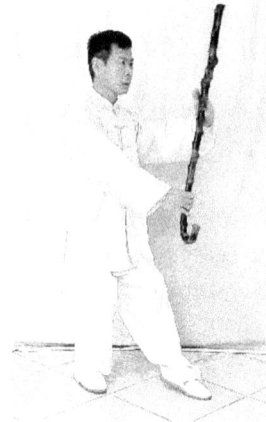

Photo 22-1

Movement 2

Hold the same stance, twist your torso left, and parry the cane in the vertical position to the left (Photo 22-2). Next, immediately twist your torso to the right as you parry the cane to the right. You can turn the left toes inward to facilitate your torso's turning right (Photo 22-3).

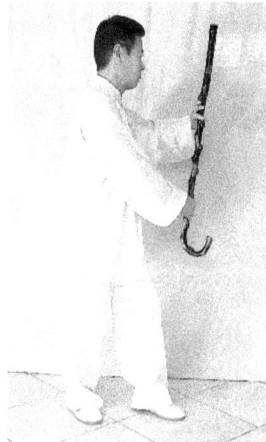

Photo 22-2

Key Points

1) Parrying left and right deflects an incoming weapon targeting your front center.

2) Use your torso's rotation to power the cane parry.

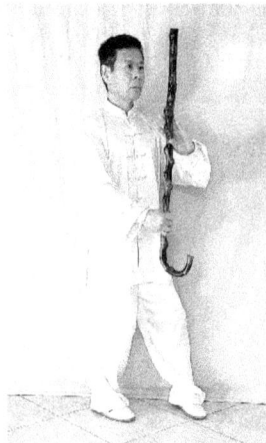

Photo 22-3

Posture 23: Turn-Around Strike 腰斬白蛇

Movement 1

Continue turning your torso to the right and step to the west with your left foot. Try to turn the left foot inward, pointing to the northwest corner. Hold the cane still and vertical in front of your chest (Photo 23-1).

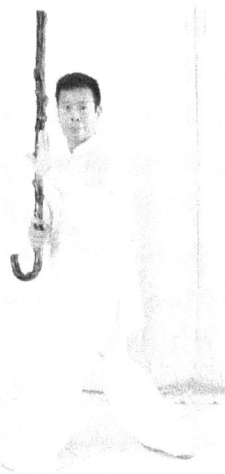

Photo 23-1

Movement 2

Turn your torso to face the back (north), and step to the east with your right foot, bending at the knee into a right bow stance. At the same time, sweep the cane to the right with the cane lined up with your right arm at shoulder height. Next, your left palm follows your torso's turning to guard at the right elbow (Photo 23-2). Optionally, release the left palm to your rear left (Photo 23-3).

Key Points

1) Use your torso's rotation to sweep the cane for a horizontal strike.

2) The optional move of extending the left arm and palm to the left rear can balance the cane as it sweeps out.

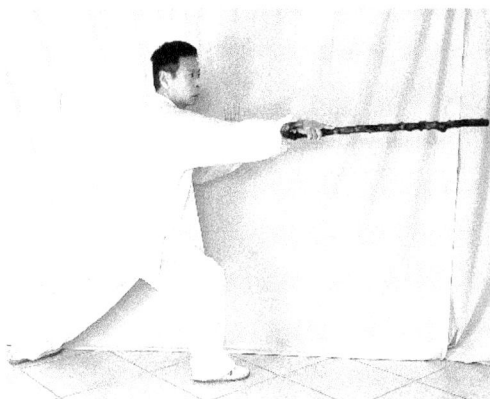

Photo 23-2

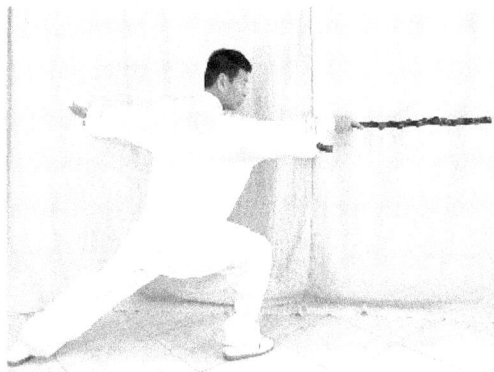

Photo 23-3

Posture 24: Dragon Swings Tail 黑龍擺尾

Movement 1

Shift weight back and withdraw your right foot. At the same time, parry the cane outside the right leg (Photo 24-1). Hold both hands at the cane handle and raise the cane above your right shoulder (Photo 24-2).

Movement 2

Whack the cane diagonally across the front of your torso to your lower left side with your left foot turning outward to the northeast. Squat down into a resting stance with the right leg behind your left leg (Photo 24-3).

Key Points

1) Use your torso's twist to the left to power the strike.

2) You can squat halfway down at the ending pose if you are not flexible enough to squat into a full resting stance.

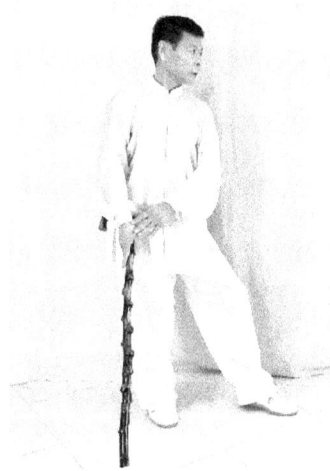

Photo 24-1

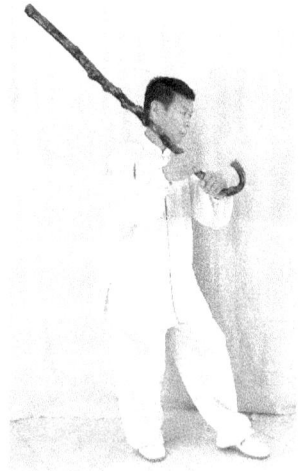

Photo 24-2

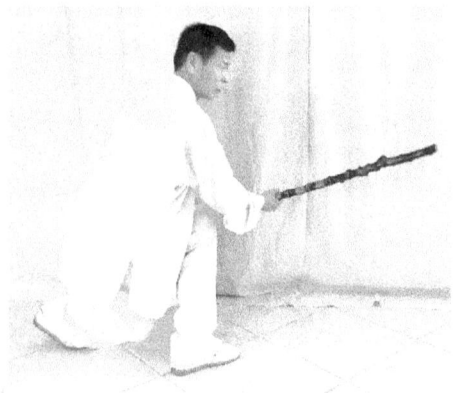

Photo 24-3

Posture 25: Head Smashing Cane 當頭杖

Movement 1

Stand up and parry the cane from outside your left and wrap the cane around the back of your head with both hands holding it above your head. Keep weight on your left foot with the right foot resting on the ball ready to step out (Photo 25-1).

Movement 2

Step to the east with your right foot and bend the right knee into a right bow stance. At the same time, smash the cane forward at shoulder height (Photo 25-2).

Key Points

1) Smash the cane onto the opponent's head.

2) Use the right foot for distance adjustment. You can leap forward if necessary.

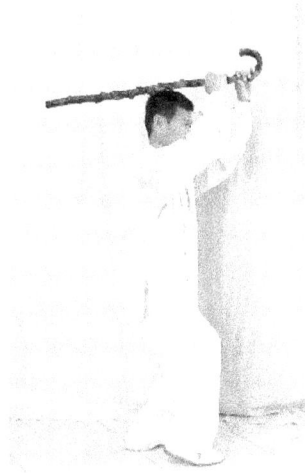

Photo 25-1

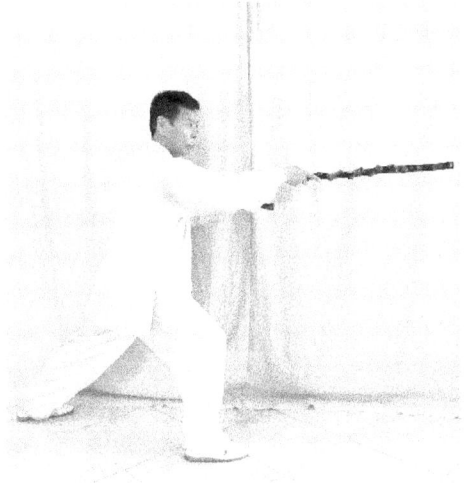

Photo 25-2

Posture 26: Lock Front Door 截門栓

Movement 1
Twist your right wrist to flip the cane in a counterclockwise circle from your right outside corner to your front center. At the same time, pull up the left foot and grasp your left hand on the middle of the cane. Hold the cane in front, guarding your chest (Photo 26-1).

Movement 2
Seeming to pause without really pausing, step to the east with your left foot and bend the left knee into a left bow stance. At the same time, bounce the cane horizontally to the east at shoulder height (Photo 26-2).

Key Points
1) Pouncing with the cane guarding in front is a move powered by your right back leg.

2) Use your left foot at the front as a brake to control the momentum.

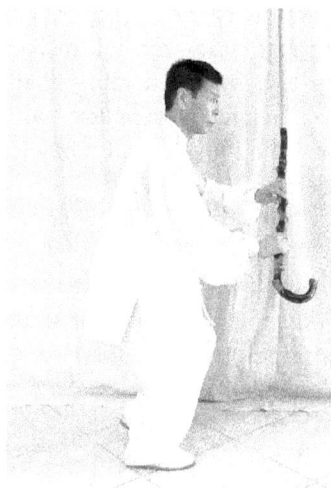
Photo 26-1

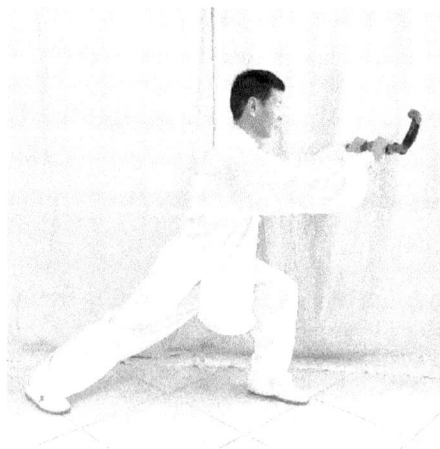
Photo 26-2

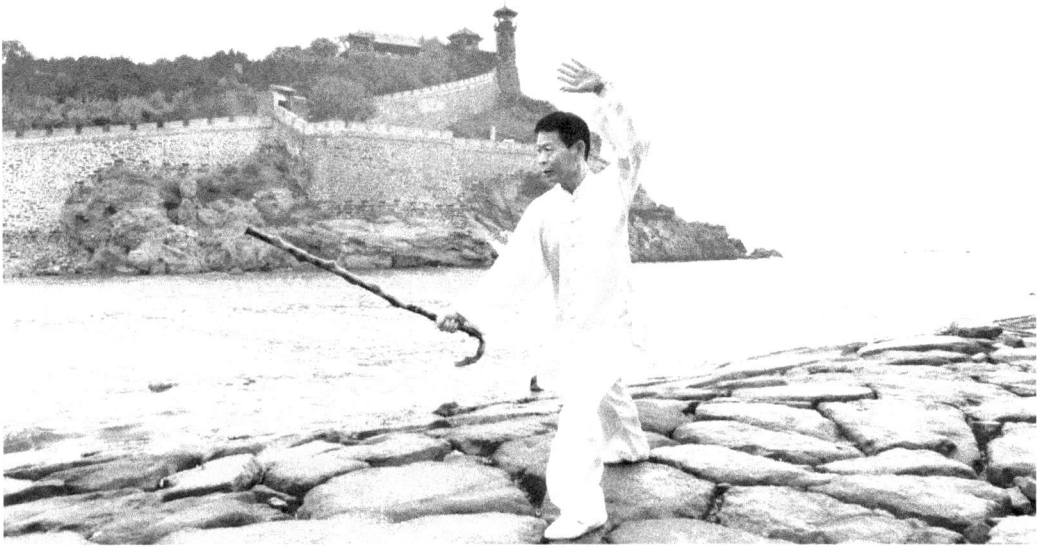

黑熊翻背

Black Bear
Turns Around

Section IV

Posture 27: Black Bear Turns Around 黑熊翻背

Movement 1
Shift weight back and raise the cane above your head as if you are deflecting an incoming weapon targeting your head. Face the southeast (Photo 27-1).

Movement 2
Turn to your right and parry the cane in a large curve from the southeast upper corner to the northwest lower corner. Lift your right knee and let the cane guard outside your right knee. At the same time, take your left hand off the cane and hold the palm facing up above your head. Look to your right (Photo 27-2).

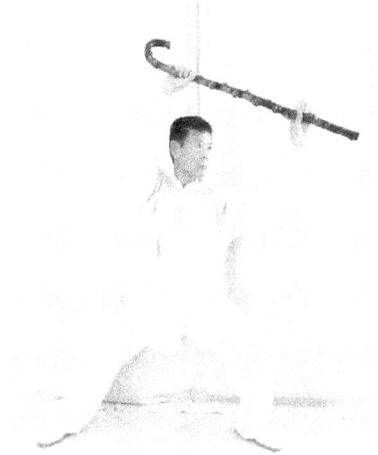

Photo 27-1

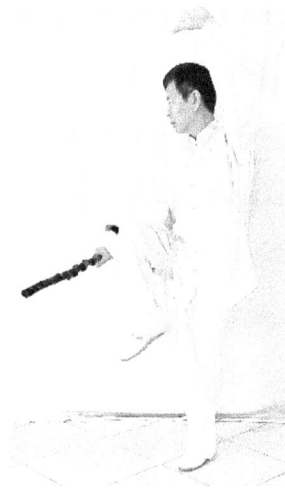

Photo 27-2

Movement 3

Turn your torso to face the back (north), and land your right foot. Immediately step to the west with your left foot, and bend the left knee into a left bow stance. At the same time, parry the cane to your right rear corner (northeast) and lower your left palm guarding in front of your chest. Look toward the west (Photo 27-3).

Movement 4

Raise the cane from the back and hack down to the northwest corner. At the same time, ward off your left palm forward and upward in front of your head (Photo 27-4).

Key Points

1) This is a posture of turning around roughly 180 degrees from your left side to your right side with the cane protecting your head.

2) Optionally, you can jump for faster action.

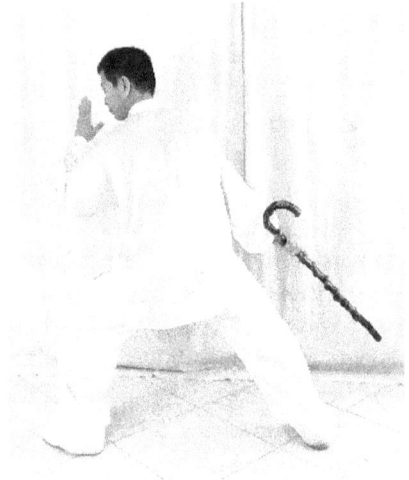

Photo 27-3

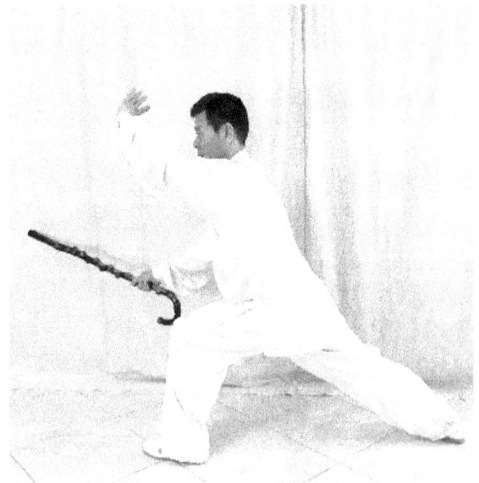

Photo 27-4

Posture 28: Lock Back Door 再截門栓

Movement 1

Twist your right wrist to flip the cane up in a clockwise half circle from your left side as if you are deflecting an incoming weapon targeting your left knee. At the same time, lower your left hand to the front of your chest and withdraw your right foot ready to step up (Photo 28-1).

Movement 2

Step to the west with your right foot, and bend the right knee into a right bow stance. At the same time, push the cane with both hands toward the west at shoulder height (Photo 28-2).

Key Points

1) This is the reverse action of Posture 26 Lock the Front Door with different steps.

2) Twist your right wrist in a different direction, and deflect the cane from low to shoulder height.

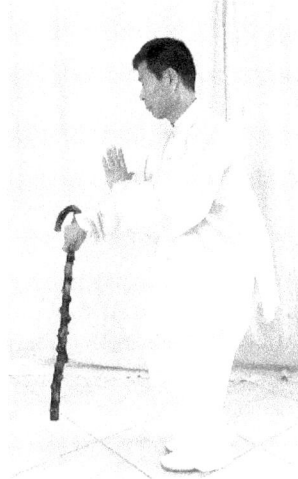

Photo 28-1

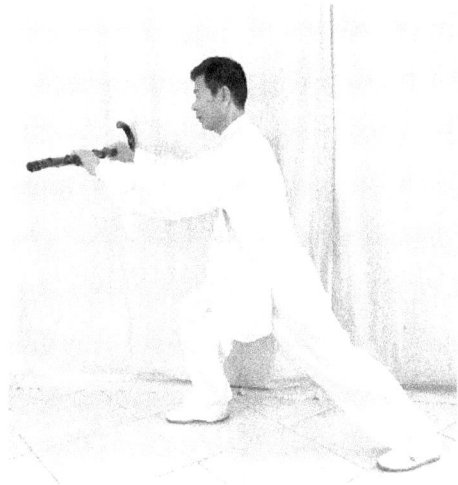

Photo 28-2

Posture 29: Heart Thrusting Cane 穿心杖

Movement 1

Turn your torso to the right and pull your left foot up to rest beside the right foot with the ball touching the floor. At the same time, parry the cane to the right and draw back the handle. With your right hand touching your right ribs, press your left palm on the middle part of the cane. Look toward the west (Photo 29-1).

Movement 2

Step forward with your left foot and bend the left knee into a left bow stance. Thrust the cane to the west at heart height (Photo 29-2).

Key Points

1) Your whole body combines power from the feet to the tip of the cane when stepping up to strike forward.

2) Make sure to line up your leg, torso, and arm in good connection with the cane.

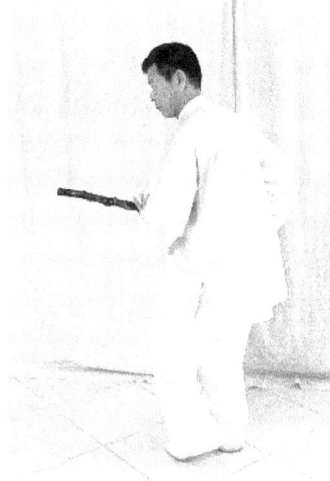

Photo 29-1

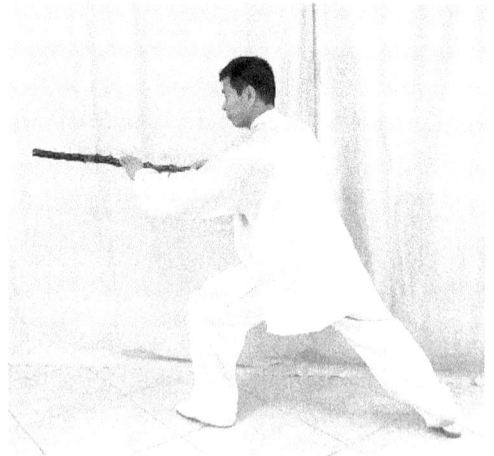

Photo 29-2

Posture 30: Waist Blocking Cane 腰攔杖

Movement 1

Turn your torso to the left and, at the same time, twist the cane to the left with the cane handle sweeping out from your right rib side (Photo 30-1).

Movement 2

Step to the west with your right foot and turn your torso to face the south. At the same time, strike the cane handle horizontally from your right rib side to the west. The sweeping strike is powered by your waist's rotation. You can stomp your right foot to make the hit stronger (Photo 30-2).

Key Points

1) Turn your torso to power the strike.

2) Optionally, you can strike the cane handle diagonally downward from your right rib side to the west by pressing your waist downward.

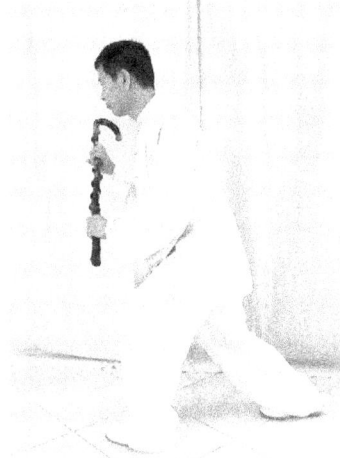

Photo 30-1

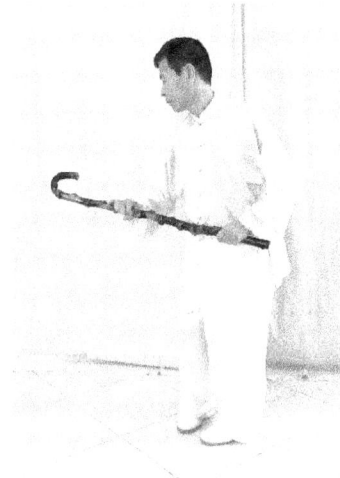

Photo 30-2

Posture 31: Crotch Striking Cane 擊襠杖

Movement 1

Parry the cane up in a counterclockwise circle from your right side across your chest to the front of your left shoulder. At the same time, step to the west with your right foot (Photo 31-1).

Movement 2

Continue the circle to lower the cane and strike the cane handle to the west at crotch height. At the same time, step a few inches away from your right foot with your left foot. You can stomp the left foot to power the crotch strike (Photo 31-2).

Key Point

Optionally, you can leap to the west to parry and strike when you need to cover a large distance.

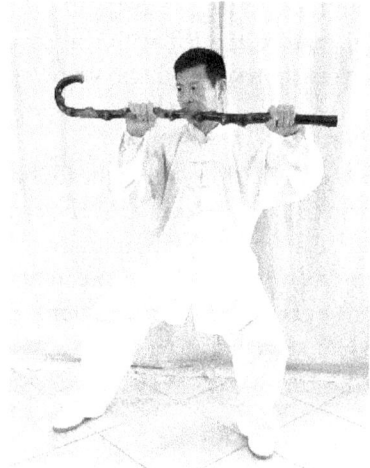

Photo 31-1

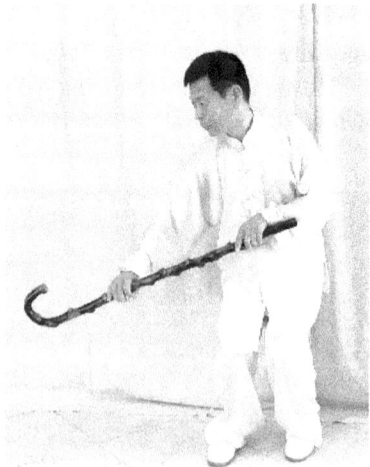

Photo 31-2

Posture 32: Head Striking Cane 擊頭杖

Movement 1

Parry the cane up in a counterclockwise circle from your right side across your chest to the front of your left shoulder. At the same time, step to the west with your right foot (Photo 32-1).

Movement 2

Continue the circle to strike the cane handle to the west at head height. At the same time, move your left foot closer to your right foot. You can stomp the left foot to power the head strike (Photo 32-2).

Key Point

1) This is the same type of strike to the west as Posture 31, but aimed at the opponent's head.

2) This posture links low and high strikes.

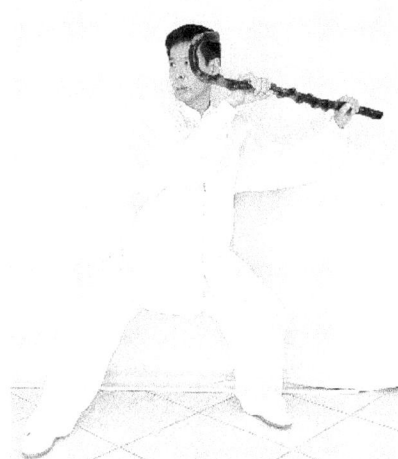

Photo 32-1

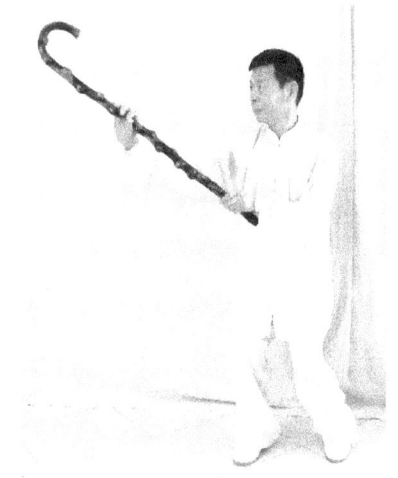

Photo 32-2

Posture 33: Dragon's Head up 翻身再舉龍探水

Movement 1

Parry the cane handle in front of your face in a counterclockwise circle and lift your right knee (Photo 33-1). Step to the west with the right foot and turn your body to the right. At the same time, lift your left foot and parry the cane down from your left side guarding outside your left knee (Photo 33-2).

Movement 2

Continue turning your body to the right and step to the west with your left foot with toes turned inward and pointing to the north. Immediately shift weight to the left foot and lift your right heel off the floor into a right empty stance. At the same time, sweep the cane in a clockwise circle to guard your head at the southeast corner (Photo 33-3).

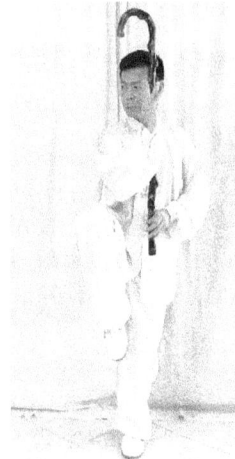

Photo 33-1

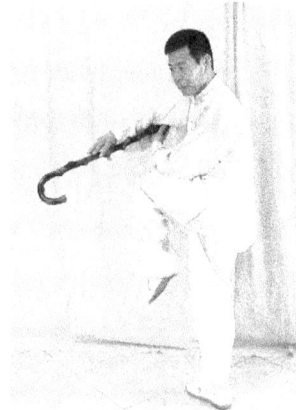

Photo 33-2

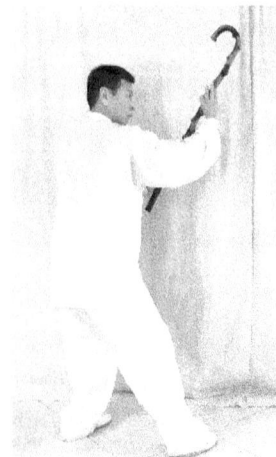

Photo 33-3

Movement 3

Lift your right foot up and parry down the cane handle to your right side (Photo 33-4). Immediately turn your torso to face the front (south), stomp your right foot, and step the left foot to the southeast corner with the cane guarding in front of your chest (Photo 33-5).

Movement 4

Shift weight forward to your left foot and bend the left knee into a left bow stance. Strike the cane tail toward the front left corner (Photo 33-6).

Key Points

1) This is a posture adapted from the Chen tai chi, long-handle big knife, *guan-dao*.

2) You can turn and jump around with the cane circling around your body like a coiling dragon.

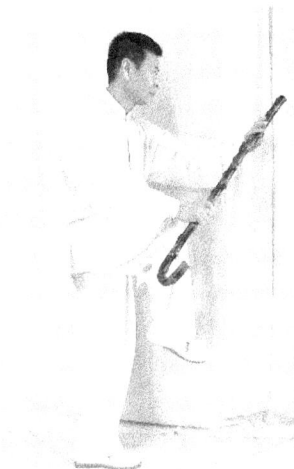

Photo 33-4

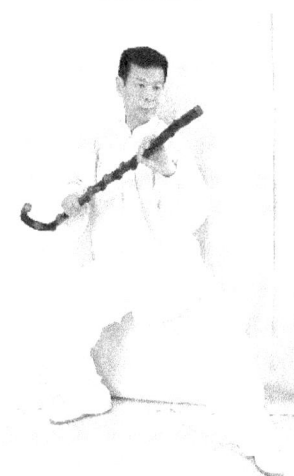

Photo 33-5

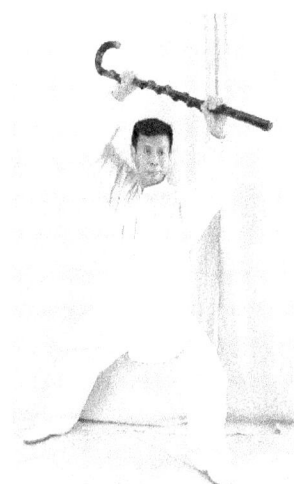

Photo 33-6

Posture 34: Dragon Coiling Around Pillar 神龍繞柱

Movement 1

Shift weight back to your right foot and parry as you wrap the cane diagonally (tail down) to your left side with the right hand above your head and the left palm guarding the right chest (Photo 34-1).

Movement 2

Turn your torso to the left and hold the cane horizontally on your shoulder. Make the maximum torso turn with the legs twisted (Photo 34-2). Immediately step to the back (north) with your right foot with toes turned inward to the west. At the same time, use your neck as a fulcrum to power the horizontal cane sweep. At the end of the turn, your left hand moves up to hold the cane with palm facing in (Photo 34-3).

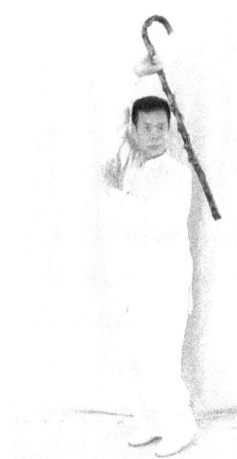

Photo 34-1

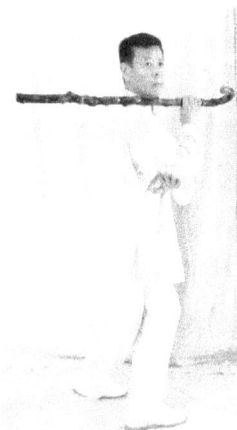

Photo 34-2

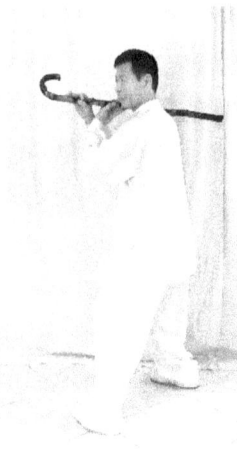

Photo 34-3

Movement 3

Twist your right foot pointing to the southwest and continue turning to your right. Face the south with body weight shifting to your right foot at the back. At the same time, your left hand takes over the cane and spins it over your head from right to left in a flat circle like a helicopter. Lower your right hand to the left rib side with palm facing down (Photo 34-4).

Movement 4

Parry the cane down across your front center to the left hip side with the cane handle pointing down. Lift your right hand to the right front of your head with palm facing upward and forward (Photo 34-5).

Key Points

1) Your body turns a 360-degree circle with the cane carried on your shoulder.

2) The cane sweeps another circle above your head powered by the twist of your left wrist.

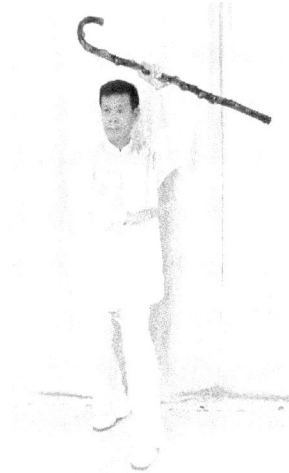

Photo 34-4

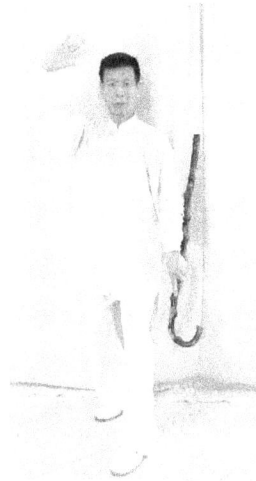

Photo 34-5

Posture 35: Wind Devil Cane 八卦轉風杖

Movement 1

Turn your left foot inward and turn your torso to the right. Ward off the cane up in front of your chest horizontally. Circle your right hand down from the right side under the cane (Photo 35-1).

Movement 2

Shift weight to your left foot and turn your torso to the right. Step your right foot to the north with toes turning outward. At the same time, take over the cane with your right hand (Photo 35-2). Without a stop, step your left foot in an inward curve to the north, and turn your torso right to sweep the cane in a larger 360-degree circle (Photo 35-3).

Key Points

1) This is an opposite circle motion from Posture 34.

2) Line up the cane with your right arm to reach a large circle sweeping hit.

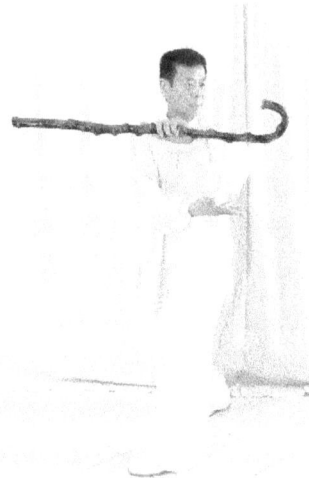

Photo 35-1

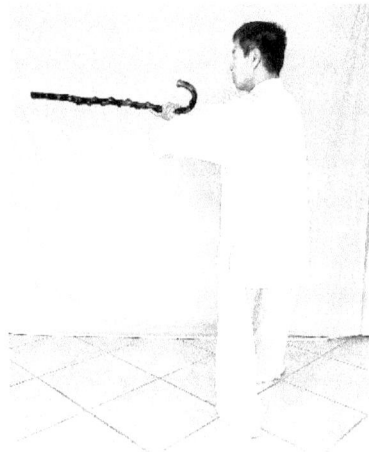

Photo 35-2

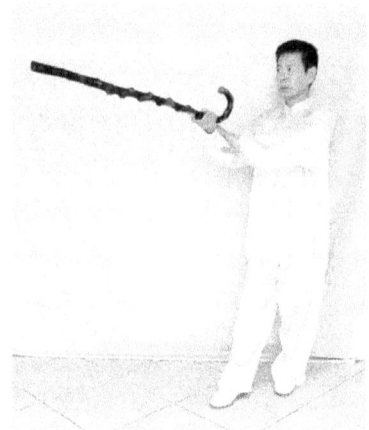

Photo 35-3

Posture 36: Closing Form 收勢

Movement 1

Parry the cane to your right side and lift the handle above your head with the tail drooping down. Wrap the cane from the outside of your right shoulder across the back to the outside of your left shoulder (Photo 36-1).

Movement 2

Lift your right foot and parry the cane from your left shoulder across your front to the outside of your right knee (Photo 36-2). Step to the southwest corner with your right foot and bend the right knee into a right bow stance. At the same time, land the tip of the cane to the floor in front of your right toes with your left palm guarding in front of your chest (Photo 36-3).

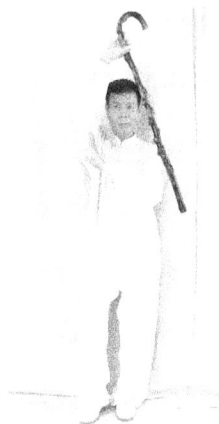

Photo 36-1

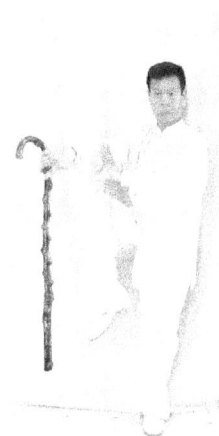

Photo 36-2

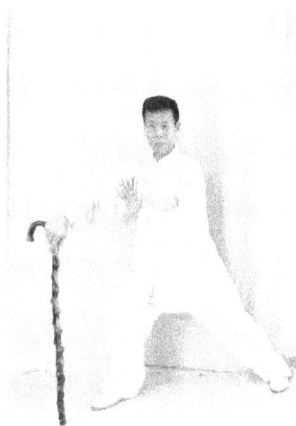

Photo 36-3

Movement 3

Unlock your left hip and shift weight into a horseback riding stance. Move your left palm in a forward curve out to the left front southwest corner. Look at your left palm (Photo 36-4).

Movement 4

Place your left foot parallel with your right foot with a shoulder-width distance, and return your left palm in an upper curve back in front of you with fingers at chin height (Photo 36-5). Pausing momentarily, drop the left palm to the side of your left hip and close in the left foot (Photo 36-6).

Key Points

1) The small circle of wrapping head with the cane is adapted to the larger circle cane sweeping momentum for soft landing.

2) The cane's small circle is also good protection for your head after the large sweeping hit.

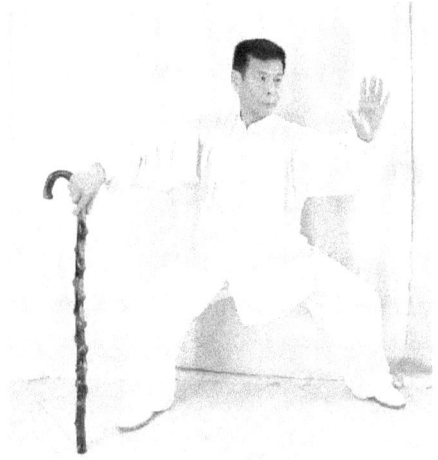

Photo 36-4

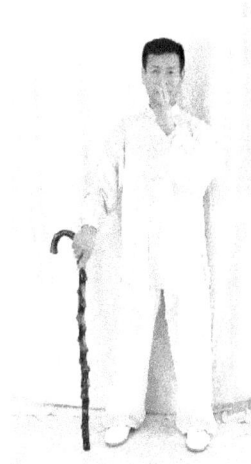

Photo 36-5

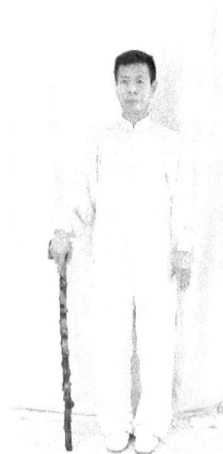

Photo 36-6

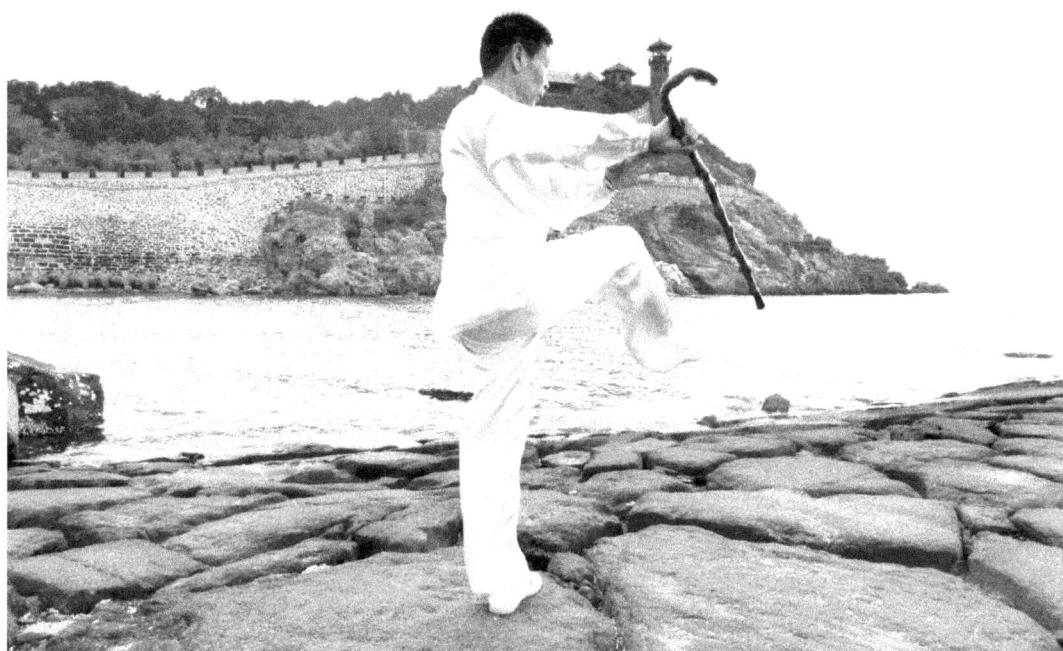

靈貓撲鼠

Cat Catches Rat

Section V

Photo series of Jesse Tsao practicing Eight-Immortals Tai Chi Cane Routine II
in front of Penglai Temple where the Eight Immortals legend originated

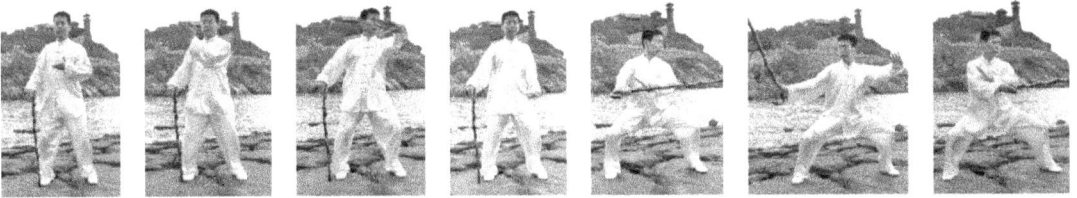

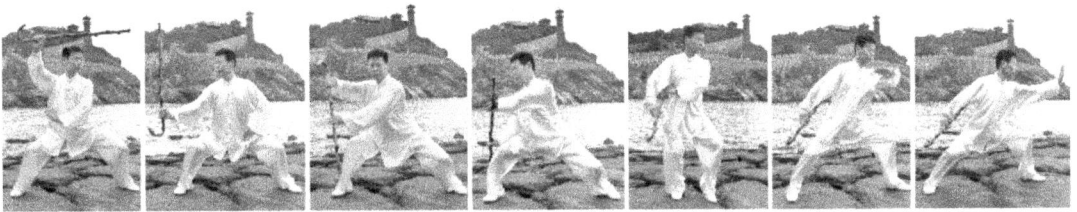

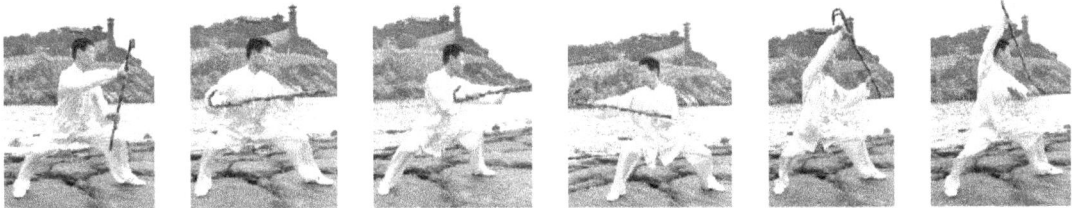

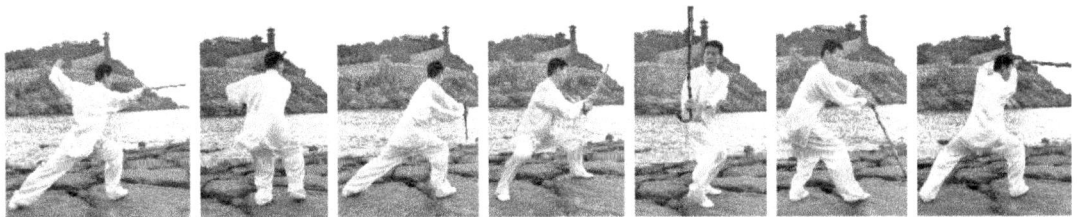

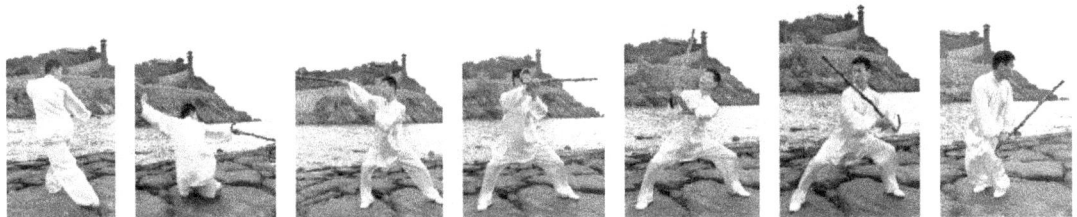

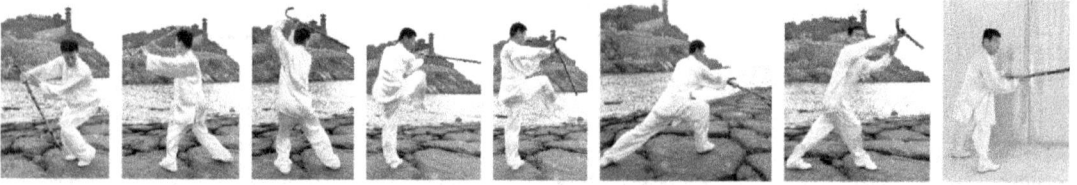

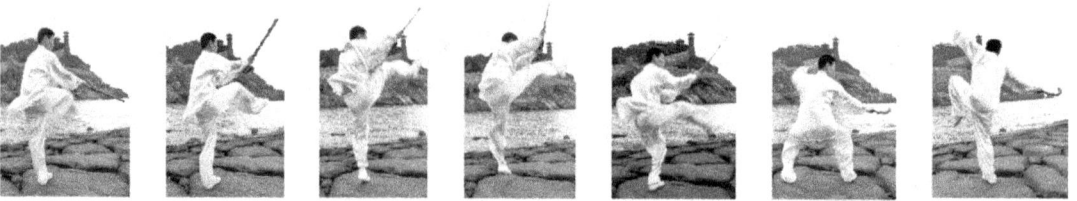

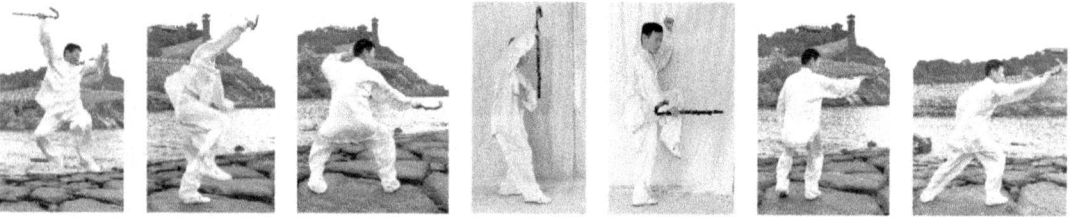

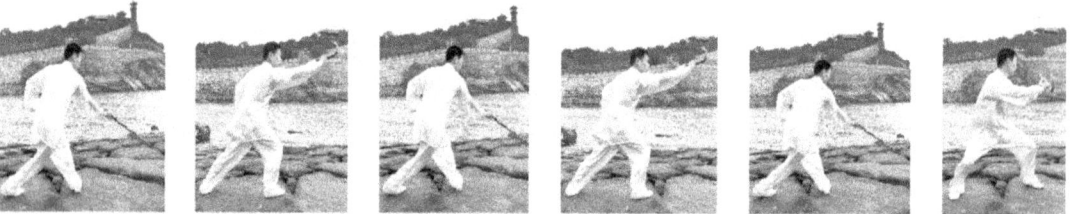

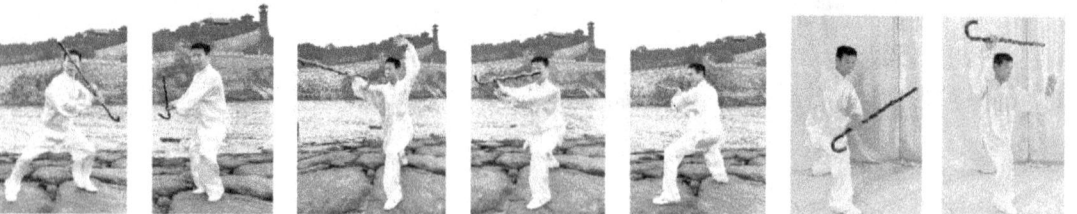

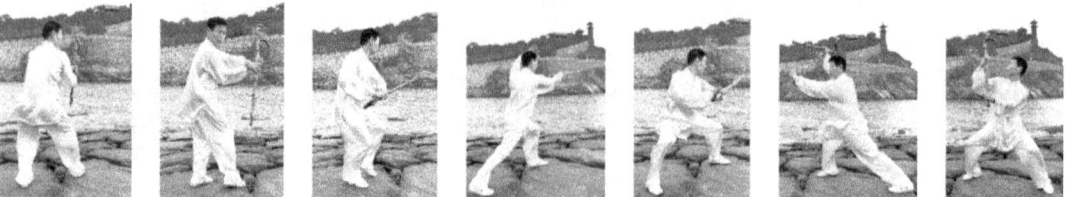

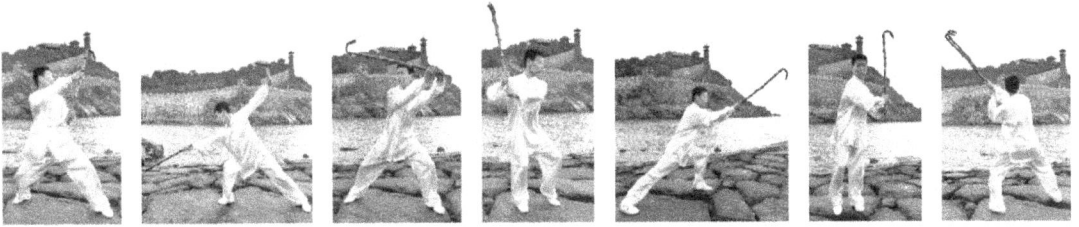

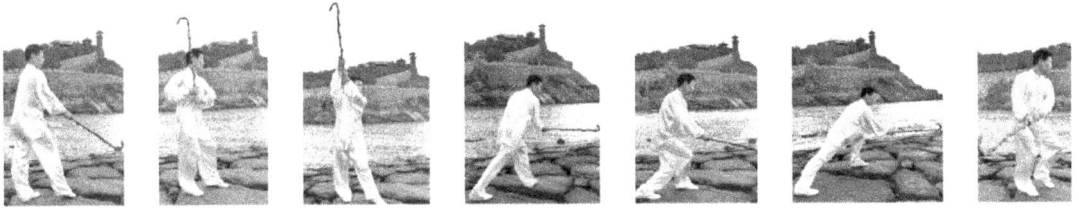

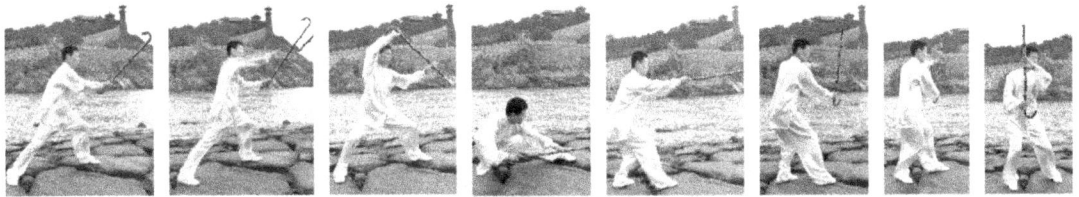

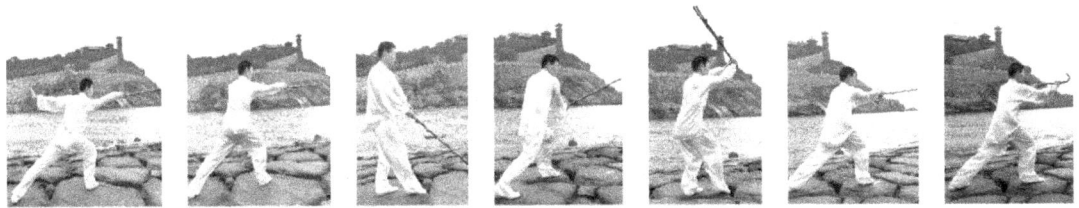

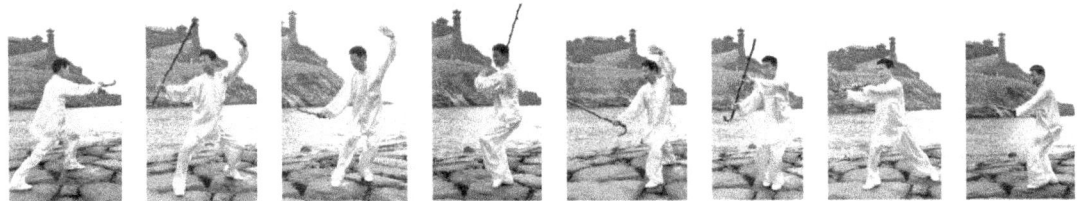

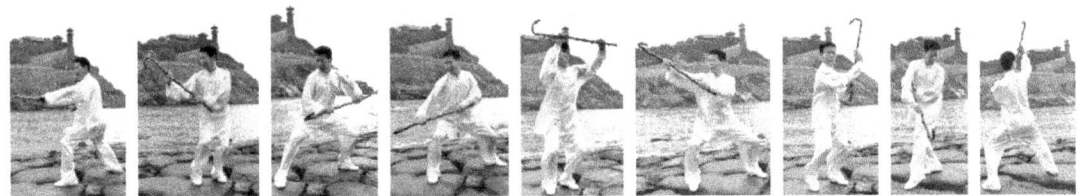

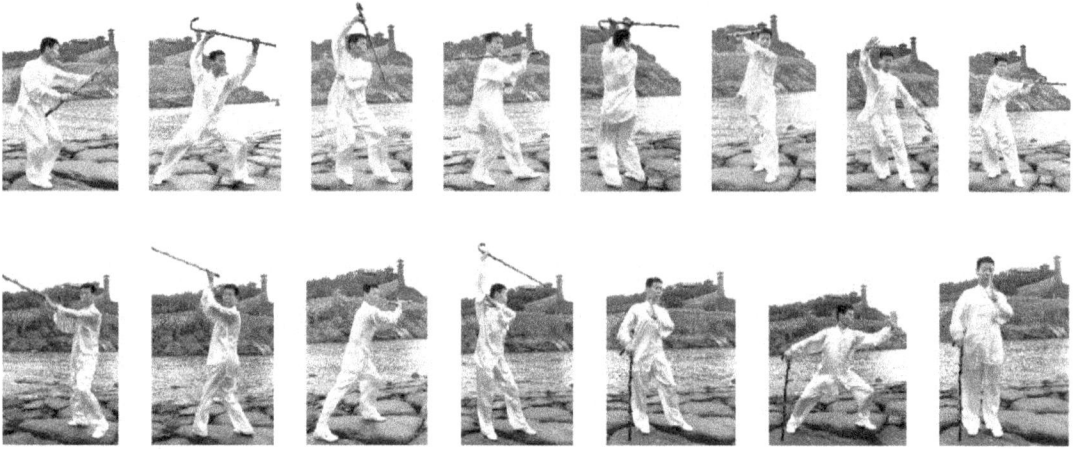

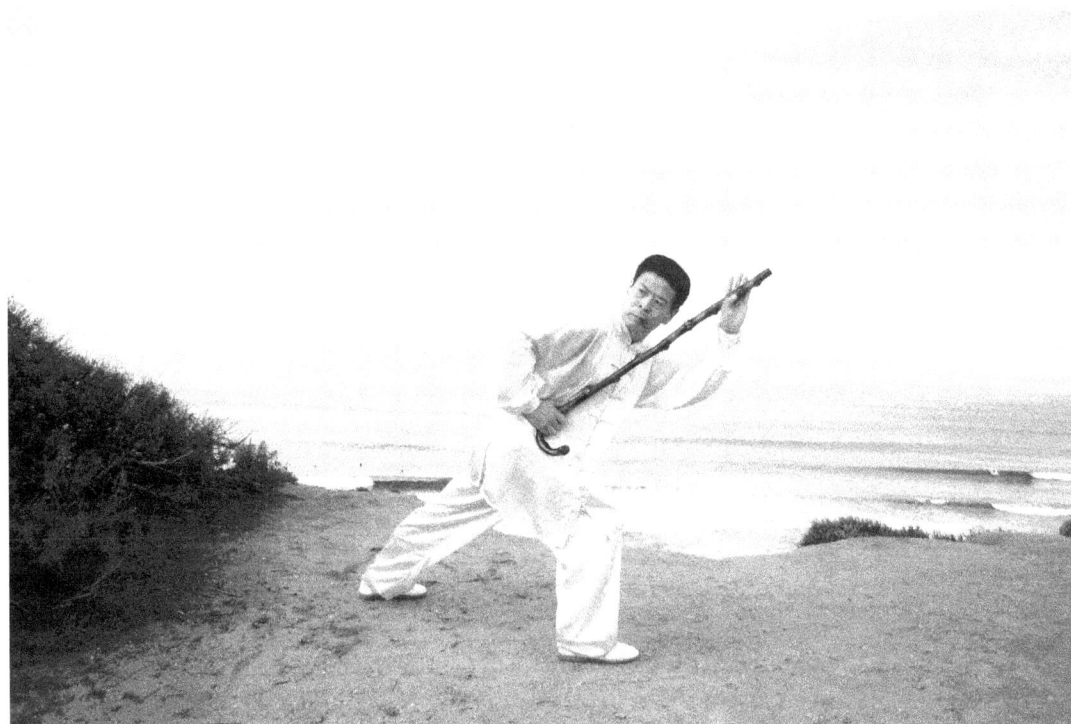

鹿回首

Deer Looking Back

Part III
Tai Chi Qigong Cane Stretch and Self-Massage

Tai Chi Qigong Cane Stretch and Self-Massage is an easy and effective preventative and self-healing exercise. It can be used as a warm-up or a seated practice (in my instructional video, I have demonstrated the entire routine on a chair). I created this routine based on my doctoral research on traditional Chinese exercise for disease prevention and wellbeing. It is a combination of tai chi, qigong, Taoist Eight-Immortals Cane, and Traditional Chinese Medicine energy points stimulation practice. This form opens the body's blockages to let energy flow, flushing out stress and cleaning out stagnation and toxins.

You may have assumed stretching was something only athletes needed to do before exercising or competing. The reality is that doing simple stretches each day can dramatically help you increase flexibility, improve balance, and relieve the pain caused by muscle and joint stiffness. Regular stretching also helps prevent life-changing falls that can threaten your independence. With a cane in your hands, imitate the different postures pictured in this book and note the key points and tips for customizing the movements to your ability. You will find cane stretch will boost your overall flexibility and loosen up tight muscles. The cane massage improves your meridian channel energy circulation by stimulating the major energy points and inner organs. It also loosens muscles, tendons, and joints. It is a simple yet powerful tool for relaxation and disease prevention. No need to identify exact locations of energy points, just use the cane to massage the area.

Posture 1: Lazy Cat Stretching 懒猫抻腰

Movement 1

Hold the cane horizontally in front of your chest with the knuckles of both palms facing down and thumbs toward the center while keeping a shoulder-width distance between hands. Your arms are bent upwards from the elbows to keep the cane about twelve inches away from your chest (Photo 1-1).

Movement 2

Open your feet slightly wider than shoulder width, fold your torso, and push the cane forward while pulling your buttocks backward to balance the arms and cane extension. Keep your legs straight and hold the pose for five to six seconds to feel the stretch in your legs and lower back (Photo 1-2). Next, unlock your knees, drop your arms, and straighten your torso. Repeat 4-6 times.

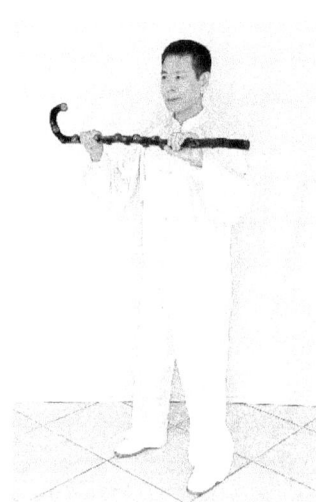

Photo 1-1

Key Points

1) This posture stretches and opens your lower back to let energy flow to clean out stagnation. The bladder meridian channel is the longest from your head along the sides of your spine all the way down through the back of your legs to your feet.

2) The degree you bend your torso forward will depend on your body condition. Ideally bend about ninety degrees, but you can take it easy and bend about forty-five degrees.

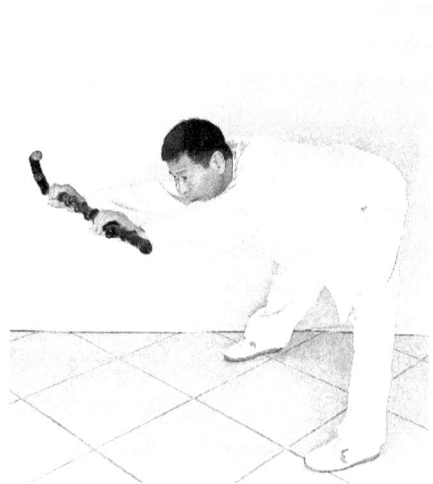

Photo 1-2

Posture 2: Hold Up the Sky 托天式

Movement 1

Hold the cane the same way as in Posture 1, lift the cane in front of your face, and look to the sky while turning your wrists up with the palms facing up and knuckles facing down as if you are lifting weights (Photo 2-1).

Movement 2

Raise the cane horizontally as high as you can and stretch your torso, especially your front chest and belly. Next, look forward and hold the pose for five to six seconds with your shoulders relaxed (Photo 2-2). Drop your arms and repeat 4–6 more times.

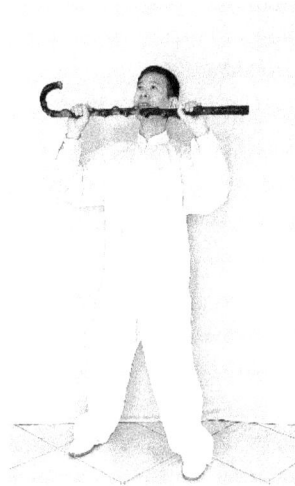

Photo 2-1

Key Points

1) Stretch the front of your torso and pull your diaphragm up to make more space for your inner organs and to refresh abdominal cavity energy circulation.

2) Optionally, you may lift your heels and stand on the balls of your feet while stretching vertically. This option will also stretch your instep.

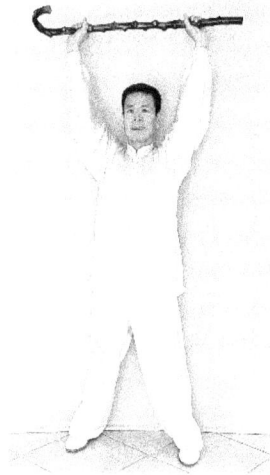

Photo 2-2

Posture 3: Tiger Pouncing 虎撲

Movement 1

Grasp the cane in both hands with the thumbs toward the center with a shoulder-width distance. Raise the cane in front of your chest, and lift one foot as if a tiger is going to pounce (Photo 3-1).

Movement 2

Step forward and push the cane forward at shoulder height with your fingers pointing up. Bend the front knee into a bow stance (Photo 3-2). Return the front foot and repeat the same move with the other foot. Step forward into a bow stance and stretch. Alternate the same move 4–6 times.

Key Points

1) Stretching the whole body's muscles and tendons releases tension. Take a smaller step without holding the knee up to challenge your balance.

2) This stretch will benefit your liver's function. Tendons are related to the liver meridian channel energy, and liver energy regulates your emotions.

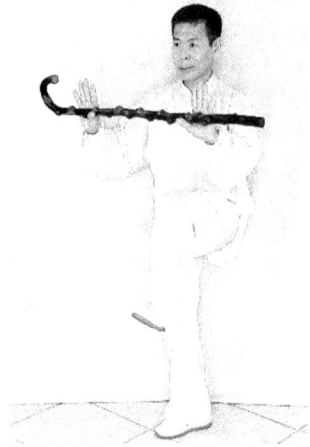

Photo 3-1

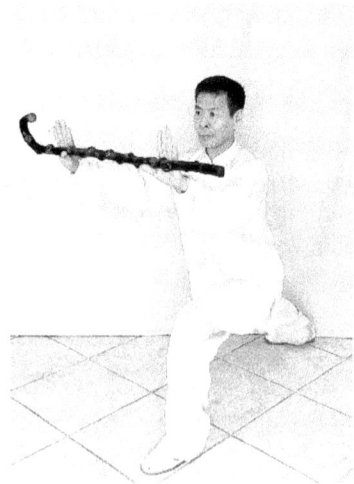

Photo 3-2

Posture 4: Deer Looking Back 鹿回首

Movement 1

Hold the cane in both hands in front of your chest with palms facing down. Step to the front left corner with your left foot, shift weight to the left foot, bend the left knee into a left bow stance, and jab the cane forward (Photo 4-1).

Movement 2

Turn your torso to the left, and at the same time twist the cane by pulling back your left hand in an upper back curve and strike forward with your right hand to uppercut with the cane butt. Keep the cane diagonally lined up with your torso, and turn your head to look at your back left side (Photo 4-2). Return your left foot and pull the cane back. Repeat the same move by stepping forward with your right foot. Repeat 4–6 times, alternating feet.

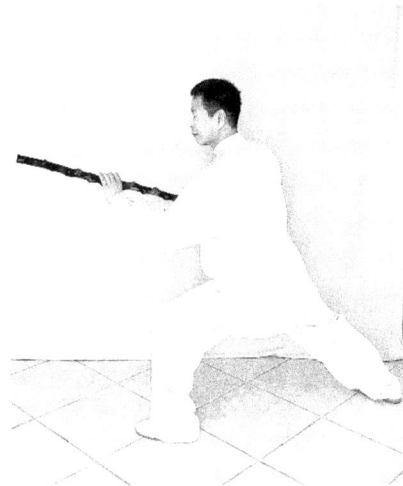

Photo 4-1

Key Points

1) This posture stimulates and nourishes kidney energy for your vitality and longevity.

2) Leaning your body forward while twisting your torso can stretch your lower back in a spiral way. You can feel this pose stretch your inner leg where the kidney meridian channel goes up from the front ball of the foot to the upper chest.

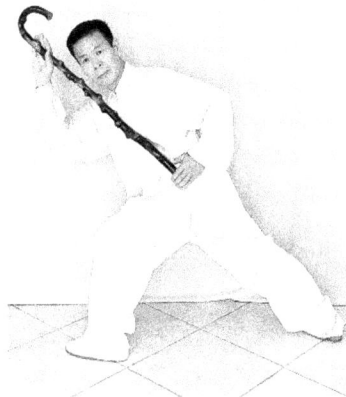

Photo 4-2

Posture 5: Open the Sky and Boundless Ocean 海阔天空

Movement 1

Hold the cane on top of your head horizontally with your hands far away from each other. Gently roll the cane on the crown of your head as if it were a rolling pin (Photo 5-1).

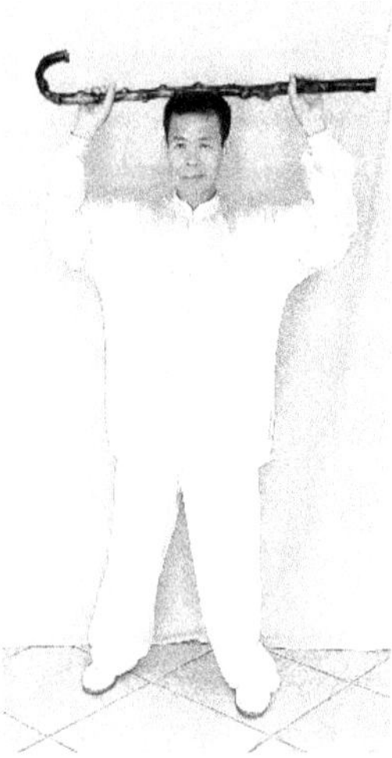

Movement 2

Roll the cane down along the back of your head and neck, continuing to the junction of your shoulders and base of neck. Bend your torso back and look up to the sky. Relax your shoulders and arms for a few seconds (Photo 5-2). Repeat 4–6 times.

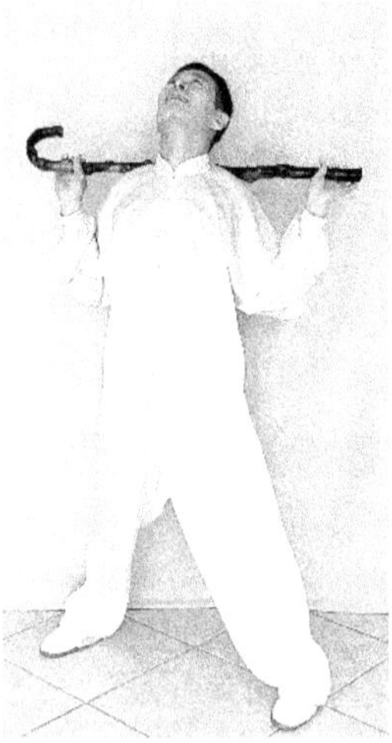

Key Points

1) Massage the top of your head, *Bai-hui* (百会穴) [GV20] to prevent high blood pressure, insomnia, and dizziness.

2) Drop the cane to the base of your neck to touch the energy point *da-zhui* (大椎穴) [GV24] to stimulate the yang energy, which prevents neck stiffness and refreshes your lungs' energy.

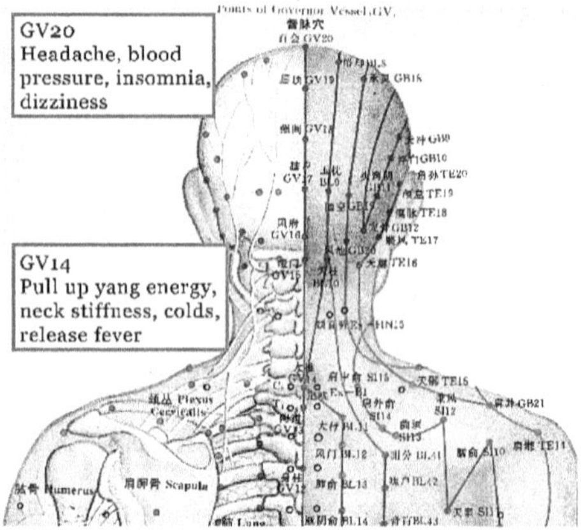

Photo 5-1

Photo 5-2

GV20
Headache, blood pressure, insomnia, dizziness

GV14
Pull up yang energy, neck stiffness, colds, release fever

Posture 6: Black Dragon Coiling Column 烏龙绞柱

Movement 1

Continue from the last posture holding the cane behind your neck, pulling down your left hand in front of your left shoulder, and raising your right hand above your head. The cane is diagonal against the back of your head between your left ear and center of your head. Gently rotate the cane to massage and pull the cane up and down a few times (Photo 6-1).

Movement 2

Twist the cane with your right hand down and left hand up to massage the right back side of your head (Photo 6-2). Repeat the move on the left side and right side alternately 4-6 times.

Key Points

1) Massaging the two energy points on the back of your head—*yu-zhen* (玉枕穴) [BL9] and *feng-chi* (风池穴) [GB20]—prevents neck pain and headache and calms your mind.

2) Apply light pressure against the back of your head. A wooden cane with natural knots will give better results.

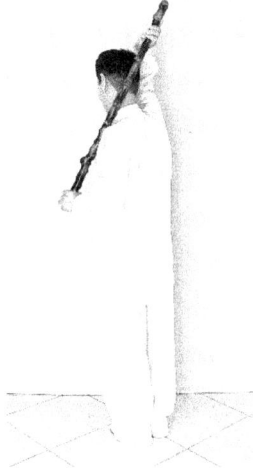

Photo 6-1

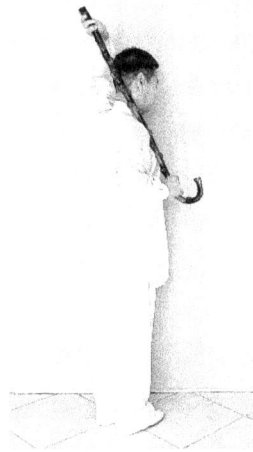

Photo 6-2

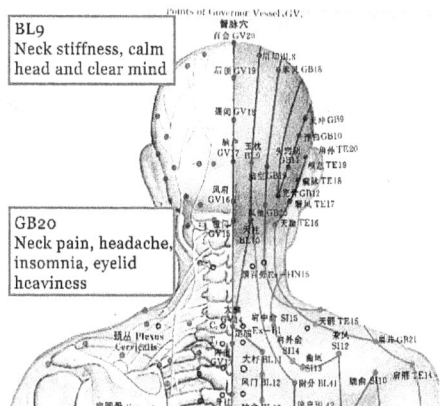

BL9
Neck stiffness, calm head and clear mind

GB20
Neck pain, headache, insomnia, eyelid heaviness

Posture 7: Tugboat 拉缱势

Movement 1

Continue from the last posture. Hold the cane on the side of your left shoulder, keep the cane handle on your back, use the hook against your upper back area between the left shoulder blade and spine. Step forward with your left foot, bend the left knee, and stretch into a left bow stance. Pull the cane forward and downward to massage your upper back with the hook (Photo 7-1).

Movement 2

Return your left foot and move the cane across your head to the side of your right shoulder. Step forward with your right foot and repeat the same massage on your right upper back area (Photo 7-2). Alternative between each side 4-6 times.

Key Points

1) This massage plows the upper back to release toxins from the energy point *gao-huang* (膏肓) [BL43], the backdoor of your lung energy. It prevents asthma, cough, and energy depletion.

2) Avoid touching your spine. The point is about 1.5 inches away from the spine line.

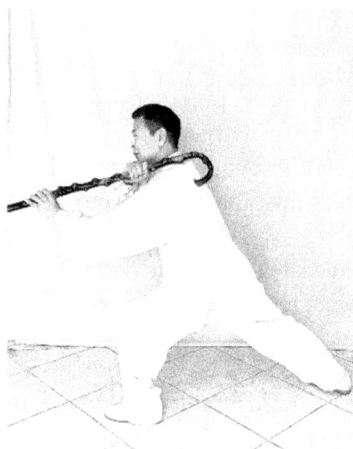

Photo 7-1

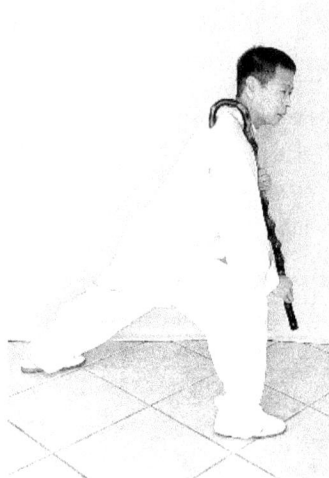

Photo 7-2

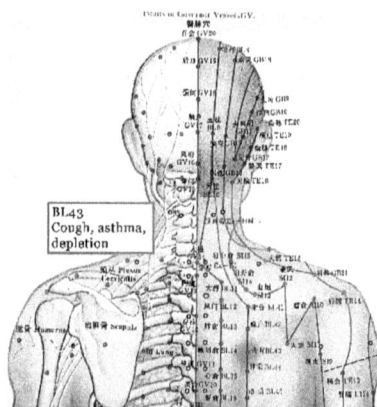

BL43
Cough, asthma, depletion

Posture 8: Wrap Head and Rub the Back 纏頭裹腦

Movement 1

Hold the cane in front of your torso diagonally with your right hand on the top above head height, left hand low at left hip level. Turn the torso to your left side and parry the cane to the left side as if you are sweeping away bad energy (Photo 8-1).

Movement 2

Circle the cane from your left side behind your back with your right hand still high. Adjust your left hand's grasp with the palm facing back (knuckles touching your buttocks). Keep the cane touching your back and rub right and left repeatedly to massage your whole back (Photo 8-2). Next, switch sides and hands with your left hand holding the hook end on the top and wrap the cane from your right side to the back of your head and rub the cane side to side.

Key Points

1) This back massage prevents muscle tightness and energy stagnation. It also stretches your shoulder to keep the mobility of the shoulder joints.

2) Optionally, pull up the top hand as high as you can and keep the cane along your spine vertically to prevent hunchback.

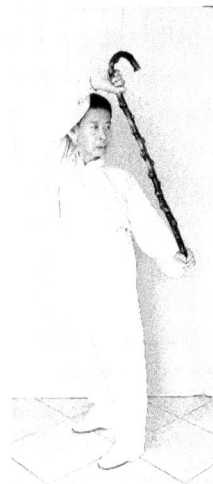

Photo 8-1

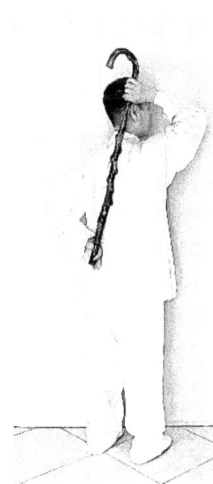

Photo 8-2

185

Posture 9: Willow Tree Bends in Wind 風擺垂柳

Movement 1

Hold the cane horizontally in both hands in front of your belly with knuckles facing out. Gently swing the cane side to side and then fold your arms in front of your chest with the right arm on top. Bend your torso forward to feel the rounding stretch on your back caused by your folding arms and the extension of your lower back (Photo 9-1).

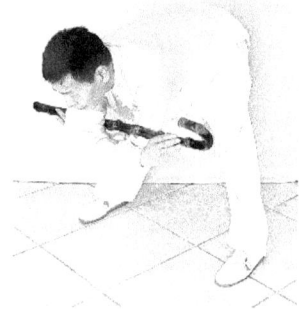

Movement 2

Lift your torso and unfold your arms. Continue to twist the cane to your right side in a clockwise circle until the cane is vertical on your right side with your left hand on top and right hand at the lower end. Fold your torso as much as you can to the right (Photo 9-2). Reverse the same motion to your left side and repeat 4-6 times.

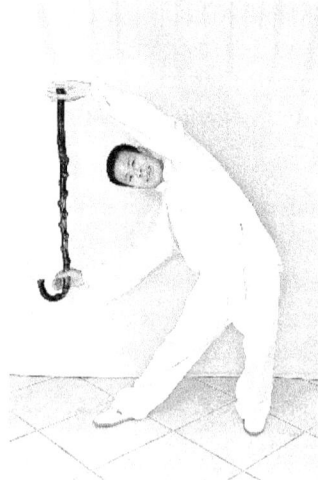

Key Points

1) Like a willow tree bending in the spring wind, this posture stretches your back and rib sides to open your body's meridian channels, especially the gallbladder channel.

2) Bending forward and sideways are limited by your body's condition. There is no need to reach too low. Stay within your comfort zone.

Photo 9-1

Photo 9-2

Posture 10: Plow the Fields 犁田势

Movement 1

Hold the cane horizontally in both hands in front of your belly with knuckles facing out. Turn the cane to your right side and use the cane hook end to stroke the right side of your waistline from the side of your spine to the front belly an inch away from the bellybutton. Next, massage the whole area around the right side of the waistline (Photo 10-1).

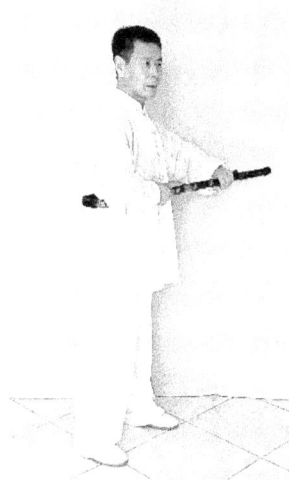

Movement 2

Twist the cane to bring the hook end to your left side. Repeat the same move on your left waist area (Photo 10-2). Alternate sides and repeat 4-6 times.

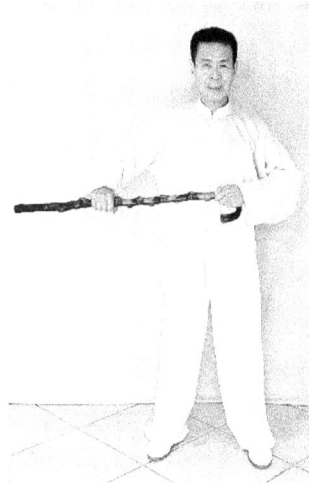

Photo 10-1

Key Points

1) Massaging the waistline can stimulate the *dai-mai* (带脉) [GB26] to reduce waist fat for weight control.

2) Massaging the side of your belly energy points *hua-rou-men* (滑肉门) [ST24] and tian-shu (天枢) [ST25] reduces belly fat deposits and improves digestion .

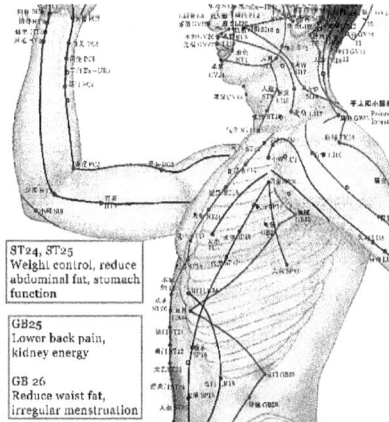

Photo 10-2

ST24, ST25
Weight control, reduce
abdominal fat, stomach
function

GB25
Lower back pain,
kidney energy

GB 26
Reduce waist fat,
irregular menstruation

Posture 11: Flat Belly 揉腹揉腿前

Movement 1

Hold the cane horizontally in both hands against your belly with knuckles facing out. Keep the hands about twenty inches apart. Rub the cane up and down against your belly and circle up to your heart and down to your lower abdomen. Move the cane up and then press the cane down with a little more force (Photo 11-1).

Movement 2

Massage the cane along your left leg, a little outside the front centerline. This area is your stomach meridian channel. Pay special attention to the middle part of the thigh muscles and three inches below the knee cap (Photo 11-2). Repeat the same moves on your right leg, and alternate 4–6 times.

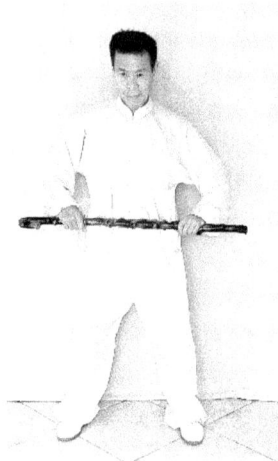

Photo 11-1

Key Points

1) Massage the front, upper belly midline energy points to prevent digestion problems, hiccups, and bloating. Massaging the lower belly prevents urination trouble or women's menstrual pain.

2) Massaging the middle thigh, fu-tu (伏兔) [ST32], prevents leg fatigue and knee pain. Massaging the spot below your knee cap, zu-san-li (足三里) [ST36], and the outside of the shinbone improves your overall well-being and vitality.

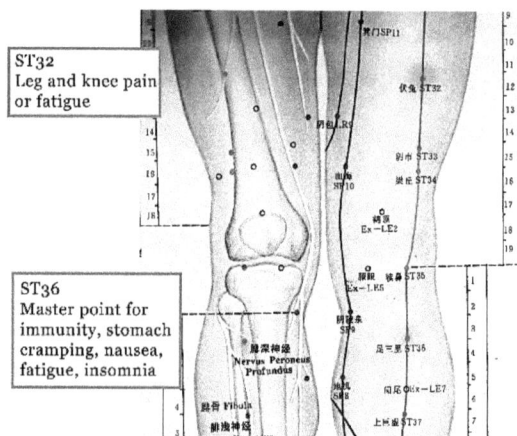

Photo 11-2

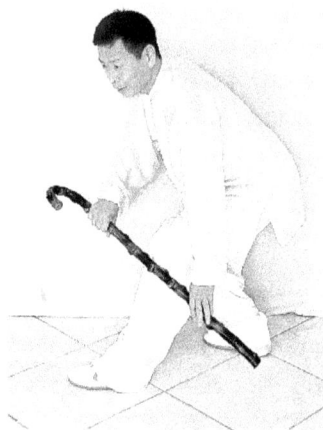

ST32
Leg and knee pain or fatigue

ST36
Master point for immunity, stomach cramping, nausea, fatigue, insomnia

Posture 12: Rowing Boat 拗臂晃背

Movement 1

Place the cane on your back horizontally and hold it with your elbows. Straighten your torso and stand for a minute. You can also move your elbows up and down repeatedly to massage the cane against your back (Photo 12-1).

Movement 2

Next, hold the cane at the same position and twist your torso to paddle the cane as if you are kayaking. Sink your hips and extend to push your shoulder to create the paddling motion. You may also paddle backward (Photo 12-2).

Key Points

1) This posture opens the chest for refreshing your lung energy. It also stretches your shoulders. When you remove the cane, you will feel a relaxed sensation in your chest and shoulders.

2) This posture will also straighten your back, pull up the *yang* energy, and prevent a hunchback.

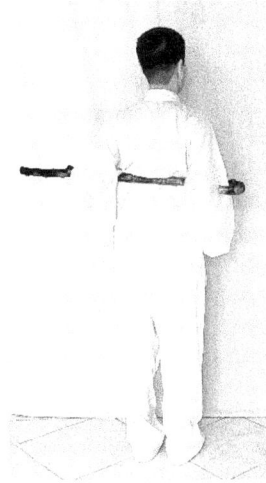

Photo 12-1

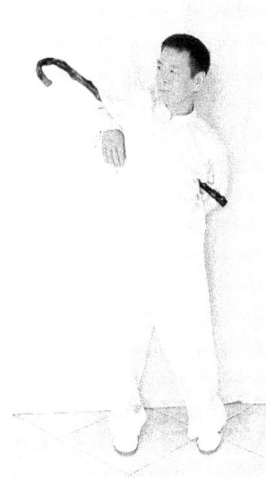

Photo 12-2

Posture 13: Flushing the Butt and Back of Leg 揉臀揉腿後

Movement 1

Hold the cane on your lower back with hands about twenty inches apart, palms facing out. Massage your lower back up and down and circle around to cover the side of your lower torso and the base of your buttock (Photo 13-1).

Movement 2

Lower the cane to massage the back of your leg down to your calf by squatting. Pay special attention to the base of the buttock, the back of the knee, and the base of the calf (Photo 13-2). Stand up, rest a moment, and repeat 4–6 times.

Key Points

1) Massaging your lower back improves your kidney function.

2) Massaging your buttock, cheng-fu (承扶) [BL36] and yin-men (殷门) [BL37], prevents sciatica and leg problems. Massage the back of the knee, wei-zhong (委中) [BL40], to prevent back pain, constipation, and leg cramps.

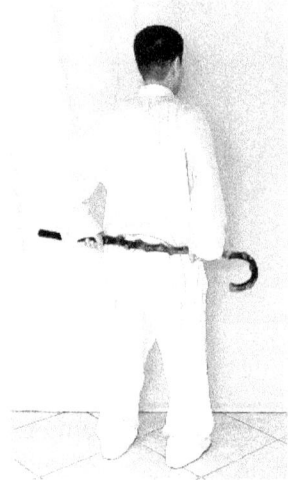

Photo 13-1

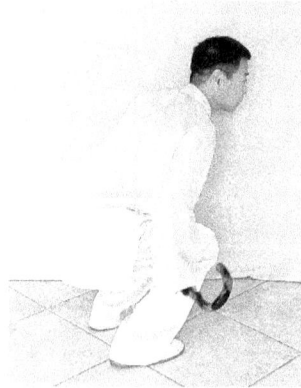

Photo 13-52

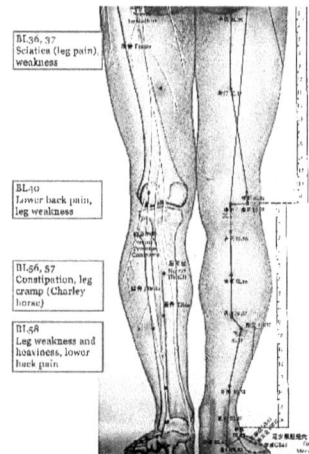

Posture 14: Kayaking 划艇势

Movement 1

Pull the cane from your back and hold it like a kayaking paddle, keeping the tip end on the left side of your torso. Use the lower part of the cane to massage the left side of your ribs (Photo 14-1).

Movement 2

Bend your torso and massage your left side down to the lower leg. Apply pressure to stimulate the gallbladder channel (Photo 14-2). Next, hold the cane on your right side and repeat the same move. Alternate left and right for 4–6 times.

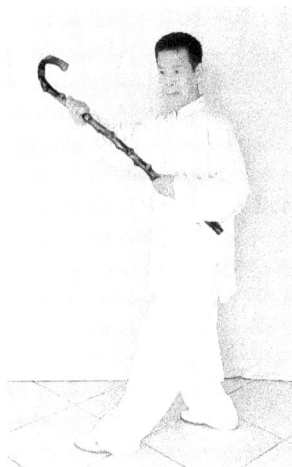

Photo 14-1

Key Points

1) Massage the rib side, *da-bao* (大包穴) [SP21], to prevent fatigue and body ache. *Da-bao* is located about three inches below the armpit.

2) Massage the outside of upper leg, *feng-si* (风市穴) [GB31], to prevent leg weakness. Massage the outside of the lower leg, *guang-ming* (光明穴) [GB37], to prevent glaucoma and increase visual acuity.

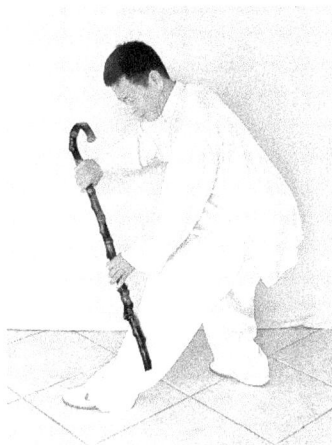

Photo 14-2

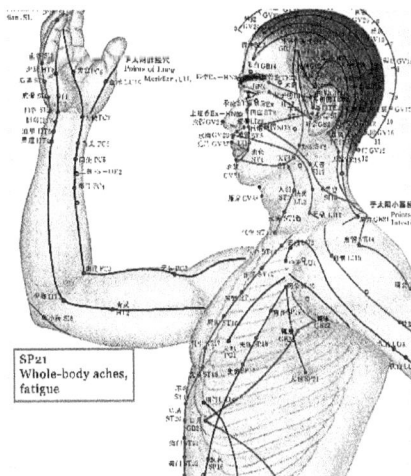

SP21
Whole-body aches,
fatigue

191

Posture 15: Hold Up Incense 一炷香

Movement 1

Hold the cane vertically with both hands in front of your chest. Relax your shoulders and chest, calm your mind, and gather your thoughts to make your heart peaceful (Photo 15-1).

Movement 2

Raise your hands above your head with the cane pointing to the sky. Hold the cane there for a few seconds (Photo 15-2) and then drop your hands in front of your belly while holding the cane vertically. Repeat two more times to finish this posture.

Key Points

1) If you practice outdoors, you can straighten your body and lift your arms as high as you can, even lifting up your heels. Optionally, for better balance, you can bend your legs a little and just stretch your torso up.

2) The main purpose is to lead your inner energy back to your lower belly, dantian.

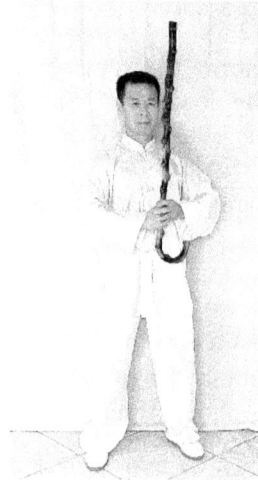

Photo 15-1

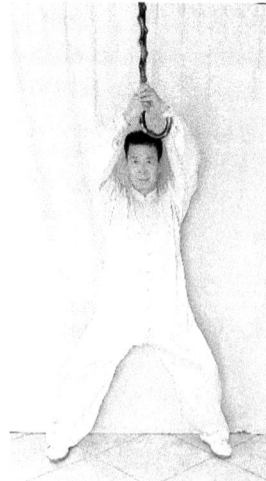

Photo 15-2

Posture 16: Closing Form 收势

Movement 1

Continue from the last posture, holding the cane in your right hand and twisting the cane by curling your right wrist to make a vertical circle in front of you with the cane. Hold the cane diagonally guarding in front of your chest with the tip up and your left foot a half step in front to form a left empty stance (Photo 16-1).

Movement 2

Drop the cane tip down and land it to the front side of your right foot. Pull your left foot back to the side of your right foot. Hold your left palm in front of your chest center, as a one palm prayer pose (Photo 16-2).

Key Points

1) Closing form's purpose is to gather in your qi and store energy in your dantian.

2) This posture will prevent energy scatter and return to your concentrated spirit.

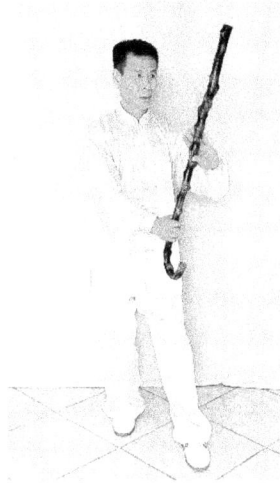

Photo 16-1

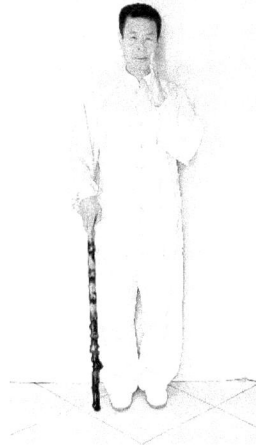

Photo 16-2

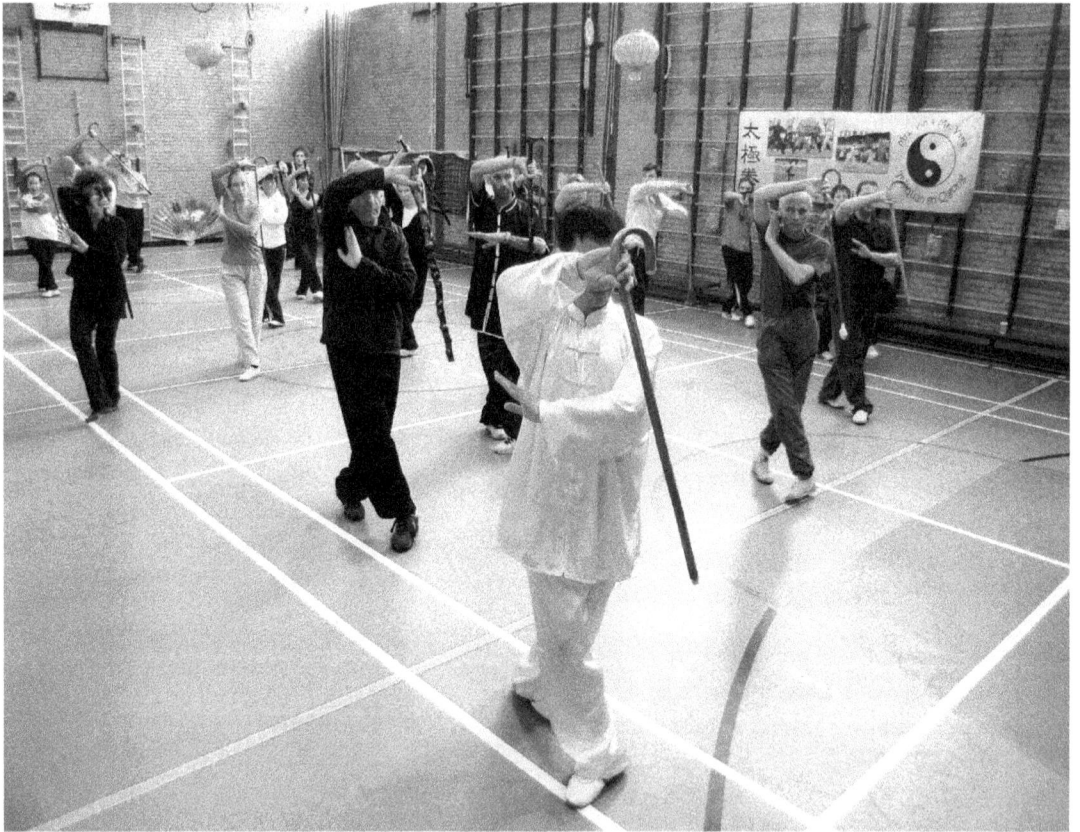

Cane Videos

Traditional Tai Chi Eight-Immortals Cane - Routine I

Traditional Tai Chi Eight-Immortals Cane is a very special Tai Chi routine. A walking cane is an everyday, common object, but is also a handy weapon in self defense! This routine is based on the characteristics of Tai Chi postures with the traditional Taoist "Eight Immortals" cane/stick martial function. It is fun for any age level to learn. Grandmaster Zhu Tiancai created the Chinese brush writing calligraphy for this routine. Detailed instruction by Master Jesse Tsao is in English with front and back view demos, as well as martial arts applications. It is a good reference for home study or a resource for instructor's teaching preparation. Suggest 30 class hours. (Difficulty: Beginner through Advanced Level). DVD, (64 minutes).

https://www.taichihealthways.com/Fundamentals-Beginners/traditional-tai-chi-Eight-Immortals-cane-routine-1.html

Traditional Tai Chi Eight-Immortals Cane - Routine 2 (Cannon Cane)

This is the answer for people looking for the martial arts aspect of Tai Chi. You will surely love the way Master Jesse Tsao presents to you this unique ancient practice. A short stick, umbrella, or any everyday object of the proper length can be used as a substitute for a cane. Like the Chen Style Tai Chi Cannon Fist, this routine is full of powerful moves and explosive strikes. Detailed instruction is provided in English, with front and back views. It is a good reference for home study, or a resource for instructor's teaching preparation. Suggest 30 class hours. (Difficulty: Intermediate through Advanced Levels). DVD-R, (62 minutes).

https://www.taichihealthways.com/Traditional/Classic/traditional-tai-chi-Eight-Immortals-cane-routine-2-cannon-cane.html

Tai Chi Qigong Cane Stretch and Self-Massage

This is an easy and effective preventative and self-healing exercise. It is a combination of Tai Chi, Qigong, Taoist Eight-Immortals Cane, and traditional Chinese medicine energy points stimulation practice. It opens the body's blockages to let energy flow, flushing out stress, cleaning out stagnation and toxins. Dr. Jesse Tsao created this routine based on his PhD research on traditional Chinese exercise for disease prevention and wellbeing. He teaches in English with side views. It is a good reference for home study, or a resource for instructor's teaching preparation. Suggested 20 class hours. (Difficulty: Beginner Level). https://www.taichihealthways.com/Fundamentals-Beginners/tai-chi-qigong-cane-stretch-and-self-massage.html

Related Traditional Forms

Traditional Yang Style Tai Chi Long Form 108

This is the most popular tai chi style. This video teaches the ancient routine of Yang Style Tai Chi Long Form 108 in 22 lessons. Master Tsao teaches each lesson posture-by-posture in English with back view and front view demonstration. There are also self-healing and self-defense applications explained throughout the teaching.

DISC 1: https://www.taichihealthways.com/Traditional/Classic/traditional-yang-style-tai-chi-long-form-108-disc-1-2.html

DISC 2: https://www.taichihealthways.com/Traditional/Classic/traditional-yang-style-tai-chi-long-form-108-disc-2-2.html

Chen Style Cannon Fist (Pao Chui) Old Frame

This is a popular routine for internal martial artists. It is characterized by spiral energy and combat techniques expressing numerous power hits (fajin). Cannon Fist is also called Chen Style Routine Two. Its firecracker power is based on the accumulated energy from Routine One's soft silk reeling. In this instructional DVD, Master Jesse Tsao presents the routine in its classic form, in English with detailed instruction and front and back view demos. He credits this video to the teachings from Grandmasters Chen Zhenglei and Zhu Tiancai.

https://www.taichihealthways.com/Traditional/Classic/chen-style-cannon-fistpao-chui-old-frame.html

Tai Chi with Baton, Bang, Stick, Staff

Tai Chi Bang: Eight-Immortals Flute

Tai Chi Bang gives you an object to focus on, making it easy and fun to gain the benefits of Tai Chi practice. This well-kept Tai Chi secret develops many aspects: Section 1 develops concentration and balance, Section 2 works on joint flexibility and arm strength, and an optional bonus Section 3 trains self-defense skill. The routine is based on characteristic Tai Chi postures with the traditional "Eight-Immortals flute" martial functions.

http://www.taichihealthways.com/Fundamentals-Beginners/tai-chi-bang-Eight-Immortals-flute.html

Tai Chi Double Bang/Baton in Chen Style

Tai Chi Double Bang/Baton in Chen Style is a practice using spiral coiling energy to power the baton's strikes. It is a weapon method rooted in traditional Chinese mace, a blunt and heavy weapon used to deliver strong smashes. This practice reinforces Chen Tai Chi's motion starting with the center dantian rotation, driving coiling energy all the way to the wrists' small twisting circle to initiate large power blows. This is unique training for wrist rotation to stimulate six hand-meridian channel's origin points around the wrist's energy flow. It will also help prevent carpal tunnel and improve arm strength. Baton length around 18" and 1.5 to 2" in diameter, prefer heavy/solid wood.

https://www.taichihealthways.com/Traditional/Classic/tai-chi-double-bang-baton-in-chen-style.html

Tai Chi Staff in Chen Style Form 36

Tai Chi Staff Chen Style is a combination of staff and spear methods and pole shaking to develop your internal strength and whole-body connection.

https://www.taichihealthways.com/Fundamentals-Beginners/tai-chi-staff-in-chen-style-form-36-new-2020.html

Tai Chi Staff in Yang Style Form 24

Based on the popular Simplified Tai Chi in Form 24, it is easy to learn for people who know the barehand form. The purpose is to use the staff to train your neigong and neijing, your internal power.

https://www.taichihealthways.com/Fundamentals-Beginners/tai-chi-staff-in-yang-style-form-24-new-2020.html

Tai Chi Ruler

This unique Tai Chi form uses an ancient tool called a Ruler which when used along with intention and breath cultivates and directs Qi throughout the body. It is a great tool to eliminate worries and release ourselves from past confusion. This beginner-friendly form concludes with a step-by-step guide on how to use the Ruler to stimulate major acupressure points on the neck, back, shoulders, and scalp, making it a fun qigong session to share with a friend.

https://www.taichihealthways.com/Fundamentals-Beginners/tai-chi-qigong-shi-ba-shi-18-forms-in- yang-style-coming-soon-2.html

Compact Tai Chi Stick Therapy

This is a therapy (or preventive practice) for people with carpal tunnel syndrome, arthritis, or Parkinson's Disease. The stick provides you with a focal point to help with hand-eye coordination. The twisting moves can stimulate energy circulation in your fingers and wrists, prevent frozen shoulders, and improve the elasticity of the tendons around your elbows. Combined with various tai chi postures, it stretches and tones your muscles, activates the hip and knee joints, improves the flexibility and strength of your spine, and prevents lower back pain. The practice is adapted from the tai chi joint locking techniques of qin-na, a traditional secret training approach for developing spiral inner energy. Therefore, this routine can also be used as a martial arts drill. DVD (60 minutes).

https://www.taichihealthways.com/Fundamentals-Beginners/compact-tai-chi-stick-therapy-new-2021.html

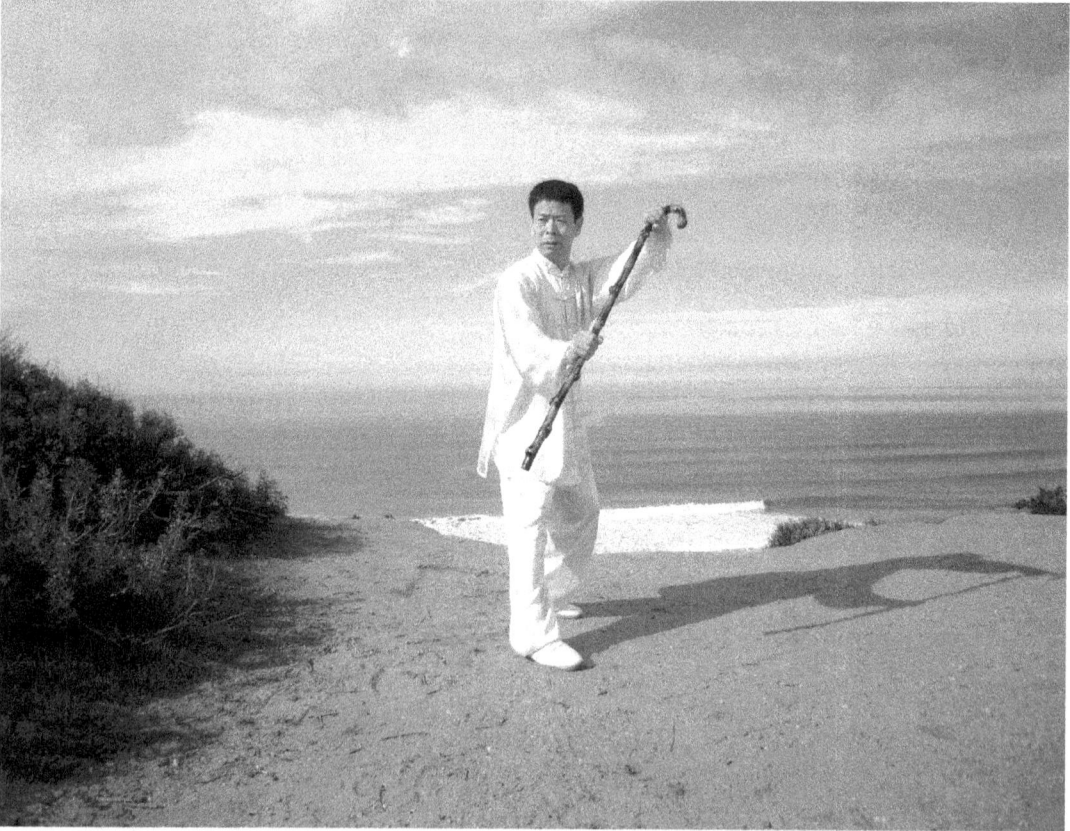

About Jesse Tsao, PhD

Born in Penglai, Shandong Province of China 中国蓬莱, Dr. Jesse Tsao is an internationally known tai chi master, qigong therapist, alternative medicine and wellness consultant and founder of Tai Chi Healthways. Penglai is known as the "Fairyland on Earth" where the legendary Eight Immortals are believed to dwell. Dr. Tsao was exposed to the rich Taoist longevity practice culture in his hometown and chose to honor his heritage with this book's cover photo of Penglai Temple.

A tai chi practitioner and teacher for more than fifty years, Dr. Tsao moved to the United States and taught his first tai chi workshop in Tucson, Arizona, in 1987. He gave up his first career as an economist in 1995 to devote more time to tai chi research and teaching. He was the chief master of tai chi for Arizona State employee worksite wellness programs from 1996 to 2015. His creation *Tai Chi Bang: Eight Immortal Flute* has been offered as a credit course by the Open College Network in the United Kingdom's Somerset Skill & Learning. His book *Practical Tai Chi Training: A 9-Stage Method for Mastery* was an Amazon Best Seller in 2021.

He specializes in the areas of self-healing, preventive therapies, stress management and mind-body wellness. Beginning his training at age seven at the Taoist temple in Penglai, his fifty years of practice include ten years of intensive study with Grandmaster Li Deyin in Beijing, China. Dr. Tsao was a gold medalist in the Beijing Collegiate Wushu Competition in 1980. He is the 12th generation direct-line lineage holder of Chen family tai chi. He has presented tai chi on a variety of national television programs and has made annual, international teaching tours since 2005. Dr. Tsao was recognized as an Ambassador for Peace and won the Hellenic Wushu Federation Honor Award, Greece, in 2018. After his twenty-one-year career as a tai chi master and health education consultant for CIGNA Healthcare, Arizona, Dr. Tsao moved to San Diego to train tai chi teachers through his rigorous instructor certification program. He has produced over 100 tai chi qigong and health-related instructional DVDs. His books have been translated into Spanish and Hungarian. His PhD is in Traditional Chinese Martial Arts Education from the Shanghai University of Sport, Shanghai, China, 2013.

Dr. Tsao's tai chi knowledge is a combination of traditional hardship training and formal academic education. His lineage shifu is Grandmaster Chen Zhenglei 陈正雷, one of the ten-best martial artists in all China, who taught him the hereditary Chen family tai chi and all weapons. He gained his practical skills directly from hosting countless seminars and workshops for other Grandmasters including Chen Xiaowang 陈小旺, Zhu Tiancai 朱天才, Li Deyin李德印, Su Zhifang 苏自芳, and Xiao Puquan 萧普泉. His doctoral advisor, Professor Yu Dinghai 虞定海, is the top-ranked, double-ninth Duan in both Chinese Wushu and Qigong. Dr. Tsao increased his understanding of traditional Chinese martial arts from interviewing and taking lessons from many experts including Abraham Liu, Dan Lee 李凯, Zang Hongxian 臧洪先, Liu Wancang 刘晚苍, Chen Yu 陈瑜, Chen Sitan 陈思坦, Xie Yelei 谢业雷, the head coach of Shanghai Sport University; Liu Jishun刘積顺, the lineage of Hao style tai chi; Liu Peijun刘培俊, the lineage of the northern Wu style; and Wu Bin吴斌, Jet Li's coach of Beijing Wushu team.

To learn more, visit *taichihealthways.com*

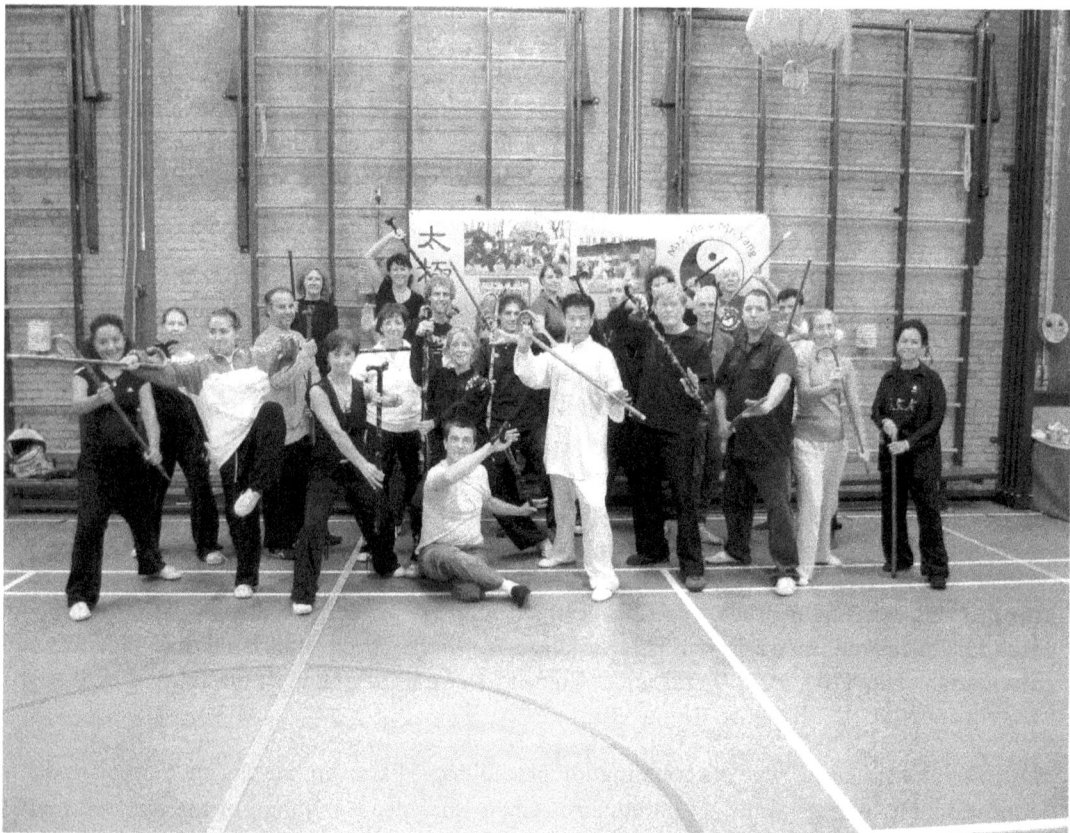

Supplement 附记

The Cane as a Weapon - Copyrighted 1912 By A.C. Cunningham

The cane as a weapon

By A.C. Cunningham
Civil Engineer
U.S. Navy

For Sale by
The Army and Navy Register
Vashington. D.C.

Price, Fifty Cents

National Capital Press, Inc
Book Manufacturers
Washington, D.C.

Introduction

The value of a cane as a weapon is the increased reach and space which it covers as compared with the hand, the great variety and diversity of motions that can be made, and the multiplication and concentration of the muscular force applied to it. As self-defense is rarely needed in these days the use of a cane as a weapon is not well known. Nevertheless self defense may be needed, and that with a cane is a quick and good one when it is understood. In these pages will be formulated a system of defense and attack with the cane which is simple, effective and easily understood, which may be aquired without the necessity of an instructor. A full comprehension of the system alone will be of use, and such practice as can be given o it will greatly increase its value. It can be made an exdcellent systematic exercise of a light and attractive nature with the satisfaction of knowing that proficiency of it may prove of material value. The work may be done in the ordinary clothing as the system would be used in actual application. An opponent is not necessary for the understanding and aquirement of the system, but where two persons can work together carefully a better appreciation of the possibilites will be had. Practice assaults should not be made without masks and padding as otherwise serious injury may result. As a system of self-defense, much or all of it may be aquired by men of advanced age, or not in especially good physical condition, and it is to those who are least prepared for defense with the hands that it might prove of the greatest value. All intricate and difficult motions have been omitted from this system and nothing used that is not easily performed and of practiacal value. In case of the system coming into use for actual self-defense it is not likely that in most cases more than the simplest and most elementary protions would be needed.

Choice of a Cane as a Weapon

This system is applicable to any cane or stick, or even an umbrella, within its limitations. In the case of an umbrella the point and butt are the effective protions. A very reliable and suitable cane for a weapon is a medium weight hickory stick, as it is of great toughness and strenght and is of low cost. A cane with a straight handle has some advantages over one with a crook or offset handle as it can be used more uniformly from each end and blows from the butt are more concentrated.

How to Hold the Cane

To hold a cane ready for instant attack or defense, grasp it at a distance about one-quarter to one-third from the butt with the thumb towards the point. This gives a balance that permits of very quick motions and allows both point and butt to brought into use. The exact location of the grasp is a matter of individual choice and the particular cane, but at least from four to six inches of the butt should project back of the hand. For close direction and control the thumb may be extended along the cane. For free swinging cuts the thumb may be grasped around the cnae. The position of the tumb is changed instantly. The grasp should be sufficiently firm to prevent the cane from slipping through or being knocked from the hand.

Left Guard

Take position with left foot and left side of body slightly advanced. Left arm raised fromthe elbow and held across the chest. Cane grasped in right hand, point down, and right arm nearly extended downward. Legs straight, or nearly so, and weight equally on both feet. The position should be comfortable and easy and at the same time alert and ready for movement. A similar left-handed guard may be used. This is the guard to use against an assault with hands. The left hand is ready to parry or strike; the cane can not be seized, but can be used in many directions.

Right Guard

Take position with right foot and right side of the body advanced. Left arm raised from the elbow and held across the chest. Cane grasped in right hand, point down and extended to the front. Right arm extended downward and to the front. Legs straight or nearly so, and weight equally on both feet. A similar left-handed guard may also be used. This is the guard to use against an assault with a cane or similar weapon. It allows a longer and stronger defense to the left guard, but less and shorter defense in the other directions, especially the rear. The right and left guards may be quickly changed from one to the other by reversing the relative position of the feet. The advantage in keeping the point down is that the cane can not be seized or pushed to one side, and it reduces parrying to two simple movements.

Double Guard, Right or Left

The general position of the body in this guard is the same as in right or left guard. The cane is grasped in both hands with the thumbs toward the center, each end projecting from the hands about six or eight inches. The hands are bent upwards from the elbows, anf the cane is held horizontally about six inches in front of the chest. This guard is used against assaults from two or more directions and may be used in place of the single guards. As blows may be delivered with either hand from this guard, it is evident that both the reach and the space are much extended. The assailant is also less certain from where to expect a blow.

Value of Attacks.

A variety of blows may be given with a cane, some of which are derived from or merge into others. All of these blows have their uses and application, and for a correct understanding they will be considered in detail.

Kind and Direction of Blows.

Jabs. Jabs are short stabbing blows given with the point or butt of cane. They are preceded by a drawing back of the hand to impart more force, and may be delivered high or low. The jab is one of the quickest attacks with the cane, and one of the hardest to avoid. Point jabs are best made with the thumb on the cane. Butt jabs may be made with the thumb on or around the cane.

Thrusts. The thrust is a stabbing blow and varies from the jab in being delivered over a longer distance and with a full extension of the arm. The hand is not first drawn back as in the case of the jab, but is extended directly forward and the weight of the body may be put into the blow. The jab and thrust are among the most effective blows that can be given with a cane as they are very concentrated and their force will penetrate clothing where a cut would have little or no effect. As a cane decreases in weight the more effective become jabs and thrusts as compared with cuts. Jabs and thrusts are also the most effective blows with an umbrella. The thrust is given with the point or long end of cane and with the thumb extended on the cane for better directing the point. The knuckles may be turned up, down, or to either side.

Upper Cuts. Upper cuts are made from downwards up, and may be delivered from the positions of guard without preparatory motion. They are not strong cuts, but are valuable as there are no preliminary indications and they are hard to parry or avoid.

Right Cuts, Left Cuts, Down Cuts. These cuts are delivered in the directions named, either high or low. They require more or less preparatory motion in the opposite direction. They are given with the knuckles turned in the direction of the blow, and the thumb may be on or around the cane. Down cuts are very strong and harder to parry than left or right cuts. Right cuts are somewhat stronger than left cuts.

Diagonal Cuts. Diagonal cuts are in an angular direction from the vertical or horizontal, and may be upward or downward, right or left. They are a valuable variation on the right, left, down and upper-cuts.

Circular Cuts. Circular cuts are full continuous swings, the first part of which is away from the object and the continuation of which is towards the object. They may be made in all directions and accumulate force during the delivery. They are valuable cuts and very deceptive, as the point of delivery may be changed without stopping the motion.

Back-handed Cuts. Back-handed cuts are made with the knuckles turned away from the direction of the blow. Upper and left cuts are most successfully made backhanded. They are not strong cuts, but may be used in connection with direct cuts and are valuable in deceptions/

Character of Cuts

In addition to their kind and direction, the character or quality of cuts with a cane are of importance and the leading characteristics will be given.

Snap Cuts. Snap cuts are short and quick and recieve most of their motion and force from the wrist. They are very qickly made and much force can be put into them. They are good cuts to use against the hands and do not carry the cane out of line.

Half-arm Cuts. Half arm cuts start from the elbow and include a wrist motion. The preliminary position will start from the shoulder, but when the cut is delivered it will be mostly from the elbow. These helf-arm cuts are of more general use than any others and may be finished with a wrist snap.

Full-arm Cuts. Full-arm cuts are delivered from the shoulder and include more or less elbow and wrist motion. They are instinctive cuts and great force can be into them. Unless there is a reasonable certainty of landing, the full-arm cut is not a good one to use. It is very plainly indicated and the slowest in delivery, and, in consequence, is more easily avoided or parried. The recovery of guard is also slower, which gives a better chance for a return attack from the assailant. Full-arm cuts may be ussed to advantage in making feints.

Swinging Cuts. Swinging cuts are made in a horizontal plane over a long arc and may be continued back and forth. Great force is not put into them until a opening may appear for landing. One of their principal uses is for keeping the distance open.

Cuts in general. In delivering a cut there should be a definitive idea of landing on a certain point where the full force of the blow will be developed. The force should be cumulative up to the objective point, and should cease as soon as possible after this is reached. Otherwise, if the blow is not landed, the cut goes wide and before control of the cane can be gained the assailant may deliver a counter attack. The force of a blow lies as much in the skill with which it is delivered as in the strength applied.

Points of Attack

The assault from an adversary, whether with or without a weapon, must be started with the hands, unless it happens to be a kick. The kick should be kept in mind and is not difficult to evade from the position of guard. A kick may also lead to an assailants defeat, as it places him in unstable balance and for a few instants he is unable to retreat. Should a kick be attempted deliver a snap cut to the assailant's shin, if possible.

As the hands are, generally, the most advanced portion of an assailants's body , they should be made one of the principal points of attack. Not only are they much exposed but comparativly light blows on them with a cane will cause disablement. Should the assailant be armed with a knife or other short weapon. his hands are all the more important as a point of attack. A pistol may even be knocked from an assailant's hand by a quick and unexpected blow.

The face, head, and neck are important points of attack. They can not always reached on a direct attack, but may be on a return attack or after a feint at some other point.

The lower half of the trunk is much exposed and is difficult to guard strongly. It may frequently reached on direct attack and is sensitive to jabs and thrusts.

The elbows, knees and shins are sensitive to comparativly light blows and may be attacked to advantage when exposed.

Parries.

In defense against a knife, cane or other striking weapon, parries may be necessary, and they are the best and most strongly made fron the right guard. In this guard the cane is entirely in front of the body and may be freely moved to the right and left. From the position of right guard with the point of cane down, two circular parried upward, one to the left, and one to the right may be made to cover the entire person. A parry should be in the nature of a counte rblow against the assailants weapon, sufficiently strong to break the force of his blow. A parry with a cane should not be made by simply holding it in opposition to a blow, as this gives the assailant a chance to divert his attack to the hand holding the cane, which the counter blow parry prevents. When the attack is made with a knife or another sort weapon the counter blow parry may be directed agaisnt the assailant's hand or forearm. Parries are the stronges when made with the thumb on the cane and the knuckles turned in the direction of the parry. The same right and left parries my be made fromthe left guard, but are more limited in their extent. From the position of double guard, right or left parried may be made with either hand, and as the cane is in a middle position, some will be down strokes and some up strokes. Thrusts with a cane may be safely parried whith the disengaged hand or arm which gives an excellent chance for a counter attack at the same time.

Return Attacks.

Having parried or evaded an assailants attack, an opportunity generally exists for a few instants when a return attack can be made to advantage. Thus a successful left parry may be continued and converted into a right cut for the head, or a right parry may be converted into a left cut. In evasions, as will be later explained under foot work, the assailant's attack is avoided by change of position, and a return attack may be made at the same time. As a general rule, return attacks have a better chance of success than direct attacks as the adversary is not in the best position for defense while his attack is being diverted.

Counter Parries.

If the assailant succeeds in parrying a cut he may attempt a return attack as described. This is met by dipping the point of the cane under the assailant's weapon with a circular motion in the direction from which the counter attack is delivered. Counter parries are the quickest made backhanded, or with the knuckles turned away from the direction of the parry. This is the position of the hand when the parried blow was struck.

Feints.

Feints are simulated or false attacks made to induce a parry, or hold an adversary in check. The feint, or series of feints, may be followed by a real attack. Thus a cut to the right may be started; if a right parry is induced from the adversary, instead of finishing the attack as a cut the point of the cane may be passed under the adversary's parry and the attack finished as a thrust. When a feint is used the direction of attack should change before the adversary's parry has touched the cane. If the adversary appears proficient in the use of feints, be careful not to over parry, and if the feints are not strong a parry may be reserved until the real attack is delivered.

Passing the cane.

One of the great advantages of the cane as a weapon is the possibility of passing it from one hand to the other and back. As either end of the cane may be used for attack or defense, this possibility of passing it from one hand to the other gives it a range and variety of application possessed by no other striking weapon. On account of this possibility it is worth while to familiarize the left hand with carrying and using the cane in alternation with the right.

Foot Work.

For the full development of the cane as a weapon of attack and defense it is necessary to be able to quickly change the location and position of the body withoug loss of balance or control. This is accomplished by movements of the feet which are executed from either the left or the right guard, and which will be described

Extend front. In making an attack to the front it may be necessary to increase the reach in order to make a hit. To do so, advance the forward foot a short distance at the same time the cut or thrust is made, the rear foot remaining in place. This advance should not be overdone for fear of slipping or losing the balance and for the further reason that the longer the extension the slower is the recovery.

Recover. To recover is to resume the position from which the movement was started.

Extend rear. The rear foot is moved back a short distance, the advanced foot remaining in place. The motion is followed by a recovery. There are two uses for this motion. First to evade an attack from the front, and second to temporarily bring one in closer striking distance to the rear.

Advance Advance the forward foot a short distanceand follow with the rear foot to the position of guard. This motion is for shortening the distance to the front. It does not disturb the position of guard and maintains a good balance and strong foot hold. An advance should be made with caution, as it may be the signal for an attack.

Retreat Move the rear foot a short distance to the rear and follow with the forward foot to the position of guard. This motion is for increasing the distance to the front. The retreat may be combined with a parry or a return attack.

Front pass. Move the rear foot in line with or slightly in advance of the leading foot, then quickly move the leading foot to the position of guard. This motion is used to quickly shorten the distance to the front by a greater amount than is covered bt the advance.

Rear pass. Move the leading foot in line with or slightly in rear of the rear foot, then quickly move the rear foot to the position of guard. This motion is used to quickly increase the distance to the front by a greater amount than is covered by the retreat. Before the second foot motion is made the original guard may be recovered in both front and rear pass.

Change guard forward. Swing on the ball or heel of the leading foot, bringing the rear foot in front to the position of guard. This quickly shortens the distance to the front and changes from one guard to the other at the same time. This motion may be combined with an attack.

Change guard backward. Swing on the ball or heel of the rear foot, bringing the leading foot to the rear to the position of guard. This increases the distnace to the front and changes from one guard to the other at the same time. The motion may be combined with a parry or counter attack.

Move right, or left. Move the rear foot in the direction in which distance is to be gained, and follow with the forward foot to the position of guard. These motions mat also be made beginning with with the forward foot. When the rear foot is moved first, the motion may more quickly be changed to a retreat.

Turn right, or left. Swing on the ball, or heel of the advanced foot to the direction desired, following with the rear foot to the position of guard.

Face rear. Turn on the balls or heels of both feet in place and face to the rear. This motion changes the guard.

Turn rear. Swing on the ball or heel of the advanced foot, either right or left as most convenient, until facing the rear, and bring the rear foot to the position of guard.

Defense and Attack.

This subject will be generally considered from the defensive point of view as one must meet whatever attack is offered. When it can be done, an attack should be recieved in front, but as it is not always possible on the start, or there may be more than one attack, defense will be considered in four principal directions.

Defense to Front

If an attack is threatened from the front, the left guard is quickly and easily assumed, an as it is not an especially belligerent position it need not precipitate the attack. All of the cuts, thrusts, and parries may be executed to the front from the left guard, and it is a good one to use if the attack is with the hands. Distance may be increased or lessened at will by foot work. The following is a odd way to meet an attack with the hands. As the assailant advances us snap and half-arm cuts at his hands, being careful that the cane is not seized. If the assailant gets within striking or grappling distance parry with the left hand and jab low at the body with point of cane. A rear extension may also be made to avoid the blow or grapple and for a firmer position. If a high grapple is made continue jabbing low at the body. If a low grapple is made raise the right arm and jab with the butt of cane at assailant's head and neck. If the assailant does not close or rush, there is a choice of attacks that can be made with a combination of the various blows and foot work. An attack on an adversary shoul be preceded by one or more feints to secure an opening.

If an attack from the front is with a striking weapon theright guard should be assumed as this brings the cane into full prominence and use for entirely covering and protecting the person. All of the cuts, thrusts and parries can be executed from the right guard to their fullest extent and advantage, and combined with foot work as to quickly secure the greatest distance bothin advance and retreat. If the assailant opens the attack, be prepared for left and right parry and evasion, and immediate return or counter atack. If the attack is with a cane it is likely to be appparent whether th assailant is familiar with is use or not. If he is not, defense is not difficult. The position of right guard invites a down cut at the head; this can be thrown off with a left parry, and a strong right return cut can be made at the same time. Every chance should be wathced for to attack the assailant's hand. Care should be taken to prevent the assailant from getting inside the guard, or effective striking an thrusting distance of the cane. Should this happen, however , change to left guard backward and jab and snap cut, seizing assailant's canw with left hand, if possible. If the attack is with a knife, the assailant's hand should be the object of short continuous attacks varied with thrusts and jabs at the body when opportunity offers. The cane should never be much out of line as the object is to keep assailant outside of the guard. If he can be kept moving backwards an opening may be made for a successful blow. If one is making a series of short advances, a very quick and long advance may be made by using a front pass combined with a frint extension.

Defense to Right.

Defense to the right from the left guard is fairly good. Right and down cuts can be made strongly. Left cuts and point thrusts are poor. Foot work in this direction is limited and the position of body is not stable. Parries can be well made. In case of closure, butt jabs can be made, or, by passing the cane to left hand, both butt and point jabs. Defense to the right from right guard is poor. Right cuts, down cuts and upper cuts can be made. Point thrusts and left cuts are poor. Parries are poor. Foot work in this direction is limited and the position is unstable; in case of a closure can be made, or, by passing the cane to the left hand, poth point and butt jabs.

Defense to Left.

Defense to the left from the left guard is poor. All cuts and thrusts are limited and not strong. Foot work is limited and the position unstable in this direction. By passing the cane to left hand, longer down, left and upper cuts can be made, and also butt jabs.

Defense to the left from the right guard is fairly good. Left and down cuts can be made strongly. Right cuts and thrusts are fair. Parries can be well made. Foot work is limited and the position in this direction is not stable. Point jabs can be made high and low, and butt jabs high.

Defense to Rear.

Defense to the rear from the left guard is fair. Down, right and upper cuts are fairly strong. Left cuts and thrusts are poor. But jabs are good. Parries are poor. Foot work is good and the position is stable in this direction. By passing the cane to left hand, point and butt jabs are possible. Defense to the rear from the right guard is very poor. Only short and weak left and down cuts, and short point and butt jabs can be made. By passibg can eto left hand the possibility of cuts is improved. The foot work is good and the position stable in this direction.

Defense in Two or More Directions.

This is a situation requiring quick judgement and rapid action. The position of double guard, left gives the most uniform reach all around, and with the cane held in both hands, ready to strike with either, there is the greatest choice of direction in which to strike or thrust. Change of location and direction by foot work becomes of great importance. The quickest change of direction is a face rear, and it may be alternatley reversed for quick action all round. The assailants must be kept from acting in unison, if possible, by attacking them rapidly and in turn. More chances of being struck must be taken for the sake of making more effective blows. Feints of cuts followed by strong jabs may give the quickest results. The most powerful jabs of all may be given with the cane held in both hands, and they may be delivered high and low and in all directions. Very strong short blows may also be struck with the middle of the cane when it is held in both hands. This two handed jabbing and striking is very useful when closely surrounded. Strong parries against the hands may also be made with the cane held in both hands, and there is the least chance of loosing it. As soon as possible get through the circle of attack so as to bring the assailants more nearly in one direction. Strike the hands of assailants whenever possible. Having delivered a blow on one assailant do not watch for its efffect, but immediatly threaten or attack another. An assault from four directions is a serious matter, but it is not as hopeless as it might seem, if quickly and skillfully met.

Special cases.

Off guard. front or rear grapple. When off guard and holding the cane in ordinary manner one be grappled in front without warning. The cane cannot then be used effectively with the existing hold. To bring the cane into play, pass it behind the body and grasp it with the other hand near the point and jab forward. If the grapple is from the rear, the cane is passed in front of the body and backwards jabs made.

*Guard agaist a dog.*A dog is wary and active and rather difficult to strike. The right guard is the most suitable with the cane well in the line of attack. Left back handed cuts may be used as feints, quickly followed by right snap cuts.

Guard with the hat. In case of an assailant with a knife a very valuable guard can be made by holding the hat in the left hand by the brim. It should be firmly grasped at the side, and can be removed from the head in one motion. The hat can then be used to catch a blow from the knife, and before it can be repeated, it should be possible to deal an effective blow or jab with the cane. In case of an attack with a pistol, a chance may occur to shy the hatt into the opponent's face and thus secure a chance to strike with the cane. The use of the hat as a guard is, of course, not confined to the knife, but it may be used against any weapon. The only disadvantage is that it pevents passing the cane from hand to hand.

Exercises.

The following exercises are based on the matter explained in the foregoing pages, and their practice will give a fuller understanding and appreciation of the system. The cuts, thrusts . and foot work, made from each guard should be first well understood . and their practice formes a simple exercise in itself. A reasonable amount of practice will make self-defense with the cane an instinctive matter, should it be needed. The exercises shouldbe done slowly at first, and the speed increased as they are mastered. Unless otherwise stated the motions are to the front. These exerciese are but a few of the combinations that can be made.

Left guard. Advance, snap down cut at the hands, parry with left hand, rear extension, jab front low, recover.

Left guard. Retreat, back handed upper cut at the hands, down cut at the heat with front extension, recover

Left guard. Back handed left cut for the hands, advance, right cut to the head, recover.

Left guard. Upper cut to the rear, pass cane to left hand, and down cut for hands, recover.

Left guard. Cut left at head, extend front and cut right at head, recover.

Left guard. Face rear, circular down cut at hands, face front, jab low, recover.

Left guard. Move right, point jab left low, turn left, upper right diagonal cut at hands, recover.

Left guard. Turn right, butt jab rear, pass cane to left hand, upper cut to front, recover.

Left guard. Front pass, start full arm down cut at head, then jab for face with butt, recover.

Left guard. Right high cut to right, left swinging cut to left, change guard forward, right high cut, recover.

Left guard. Change guard backward, snap cut at shin, thrust front low, front extension, recover.

Left guard. Extend rear, parry down cut at the head with right parry, continue as a left diagonal cut at the head, recover.

Right guard. Parry right high, left high, right diagonal down cut at head, recover.

Right guard. Down snap cut at hand, continue as a circular half-arm down cut at head, thrust low with front extension, recover.

Right guard. Start full-arm down cut, parry thrust with left hand, change guard forward, jab at face with butt, recover.

Right guard. Half arm cut at head, thrust low with front extension, recover.

Right guard. Back-handed upper cut at hand, snap down cut at head with front extension, recover.

Right guard. Face rear, pass cane, left cut ar head, face front, jab front low with left hand, recover.

Right guard. Cut right hig, parry left high, return right cut, recover.

Right guard. Advance, half arm right cut at hand, rear pass and parry left high, thrust front high with front extension.

Right guard. Thrust low with front extension, parry right high and recover.

Right guard. Change guard backward with rear extension, pass cane, upper cut forward, change guard backward, pass cane, recover.

Right guard. Cut left high, counter parry right, down cut at head with front extension, recover.

Right guard. Turn rear with swinging right cut, front pass with circular down cut ar head, recover.

Double guard, left. Cut left with the left hand, turn right, cut right with right hand, jab left with point, circular down cut to right, turn rear, right cut, recover.

Double guard, left. Left high cut to front with right hand, continue as swinging left cut to rear, continue as low point jab to left, continue as circular down cut to right, recover.

Double guard, left. Front pass, right hand upper cut to rear, continue as circular down cut to front, pass cane, cut to left, cut to right, recover.

Double guard, left. Downward cut to front, right hand, face rear with swinging right cut, face front with swingign left cut, recover.

Double guard, left. With both hands, jab front with the point high, jab rear with the butt low, jab left with the point low, jab right with the butt high.

Double guard, left. Change guard backwards, cut left to the rear with left hand, pass cane, change guard backwards, cut right to the rear with right hand, recover.

Double guard, right. WIth both hands, jab right with the butt, strike front with the point, jab rear with the point, strike left with the butt, recover.

Double guard, right. With both hands, jab front, rear, right, left, recover.

Double guard, right. With both hands, strike left with th emiddle of cane, parry downwards to the front with middle of the cane, strike left with the butt, recover.

Double guard, right. With both hands, advance and jab front with the butt, face rear and jab rear with the point, turn left and cut left with left hand, pass cane , cut right to rear, recover.

Double guard, right. Swinging cut to right with right hand, and back to guard, face rear, swingign cut to left with left hand, and back to guard, repeat.

Double guard, right. With right hand, upper cut to front, continue as a circular down cut to rear, continue as upper cut to left, continue as curcular down cut to right, recover.

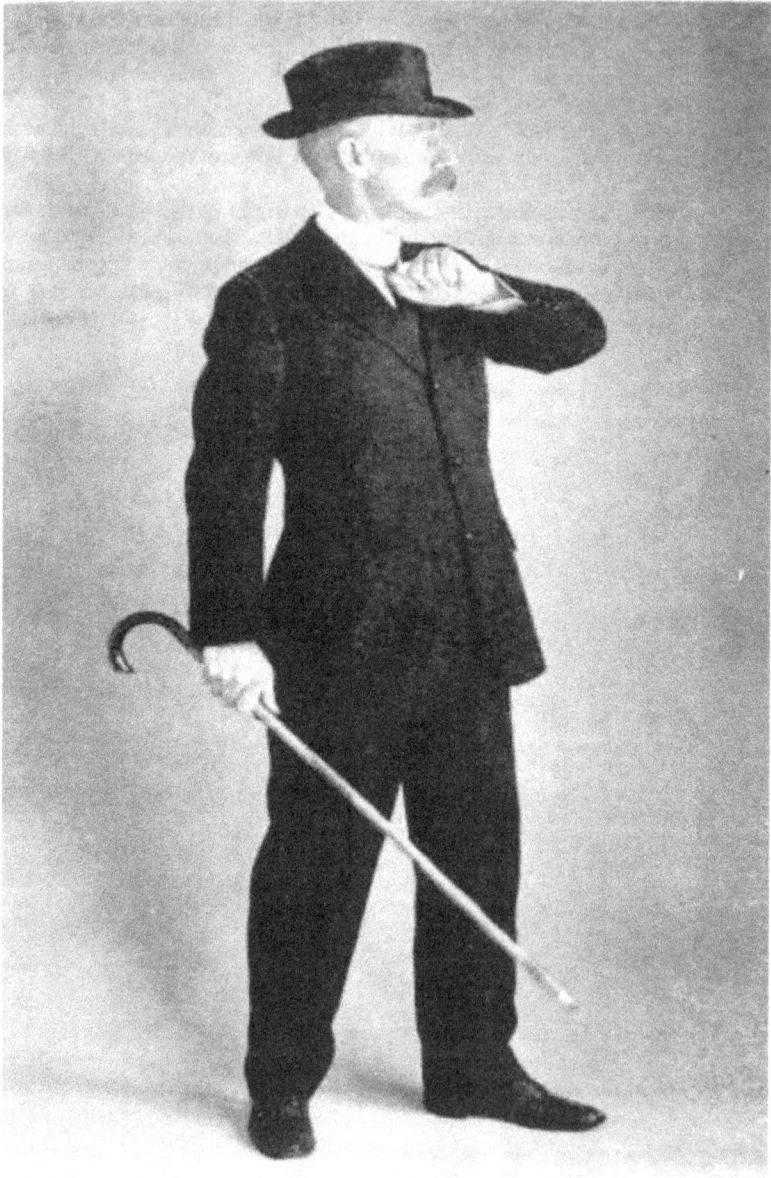

Left guard.

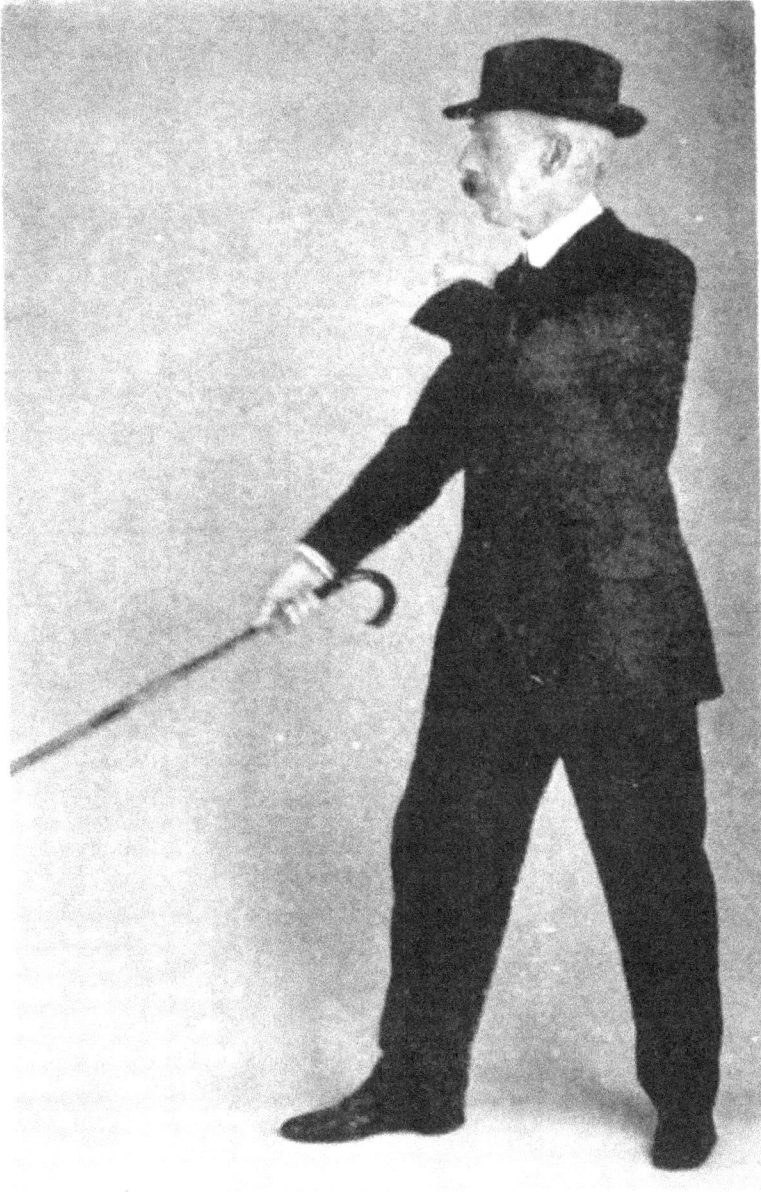

Right guard.

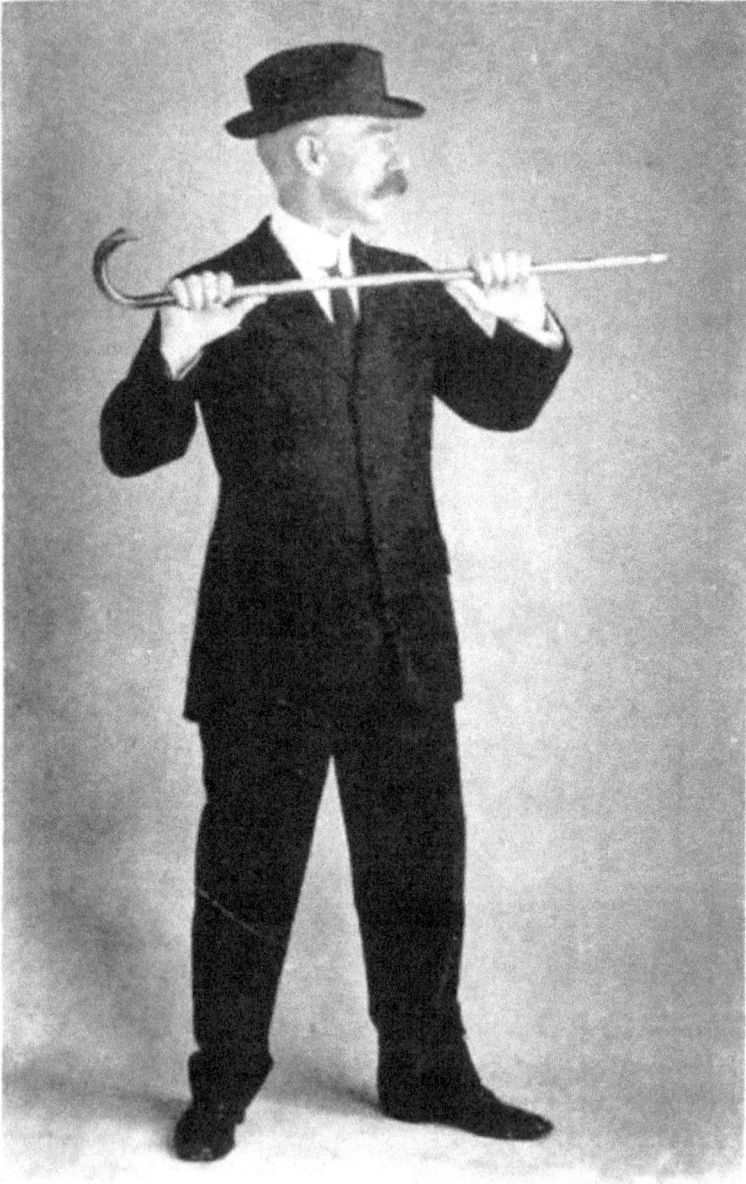

Double guard, left.

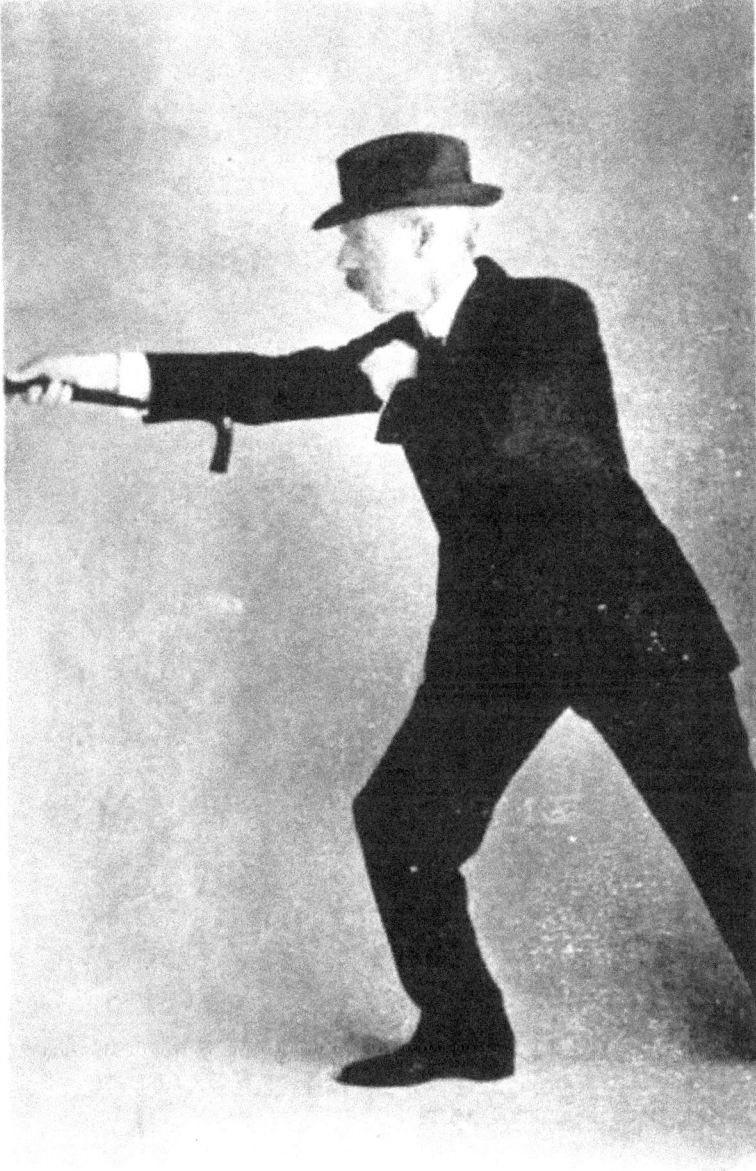

*From right guard, thrust front, with
front extension.*

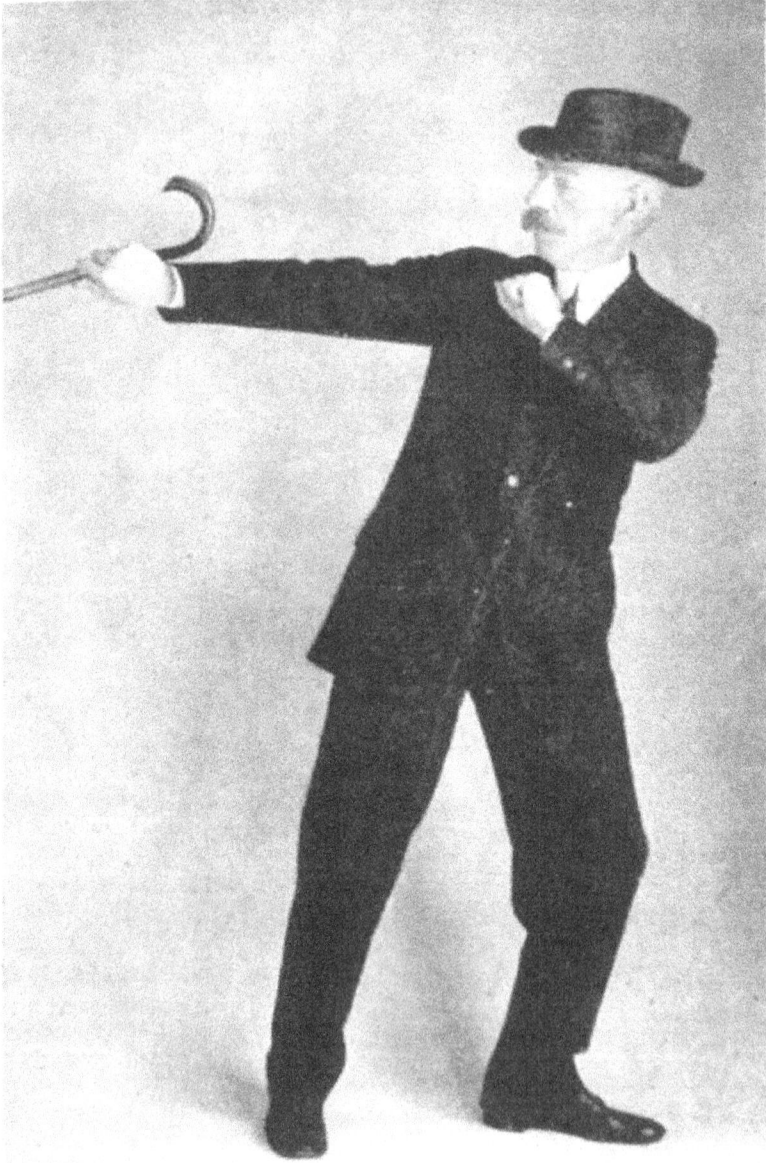

From left guard, upper cut to rear.

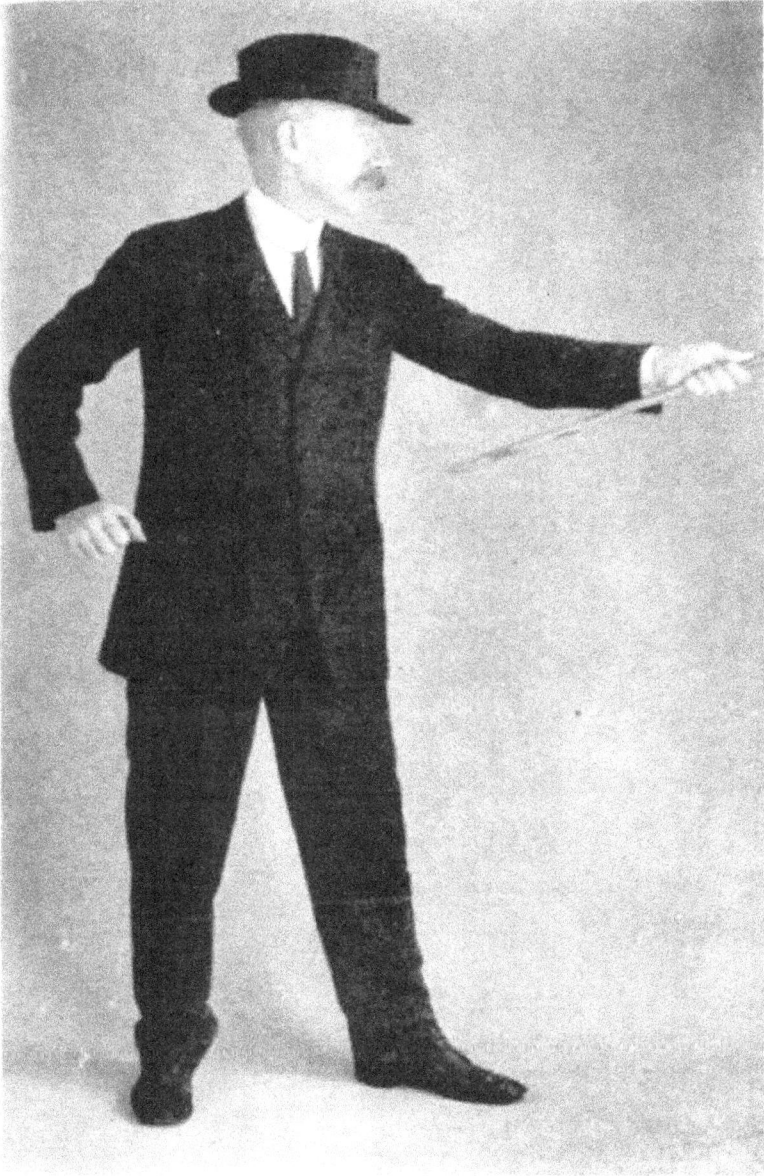

*From left guard, pass cane to left hand
and circular down cut to front.*

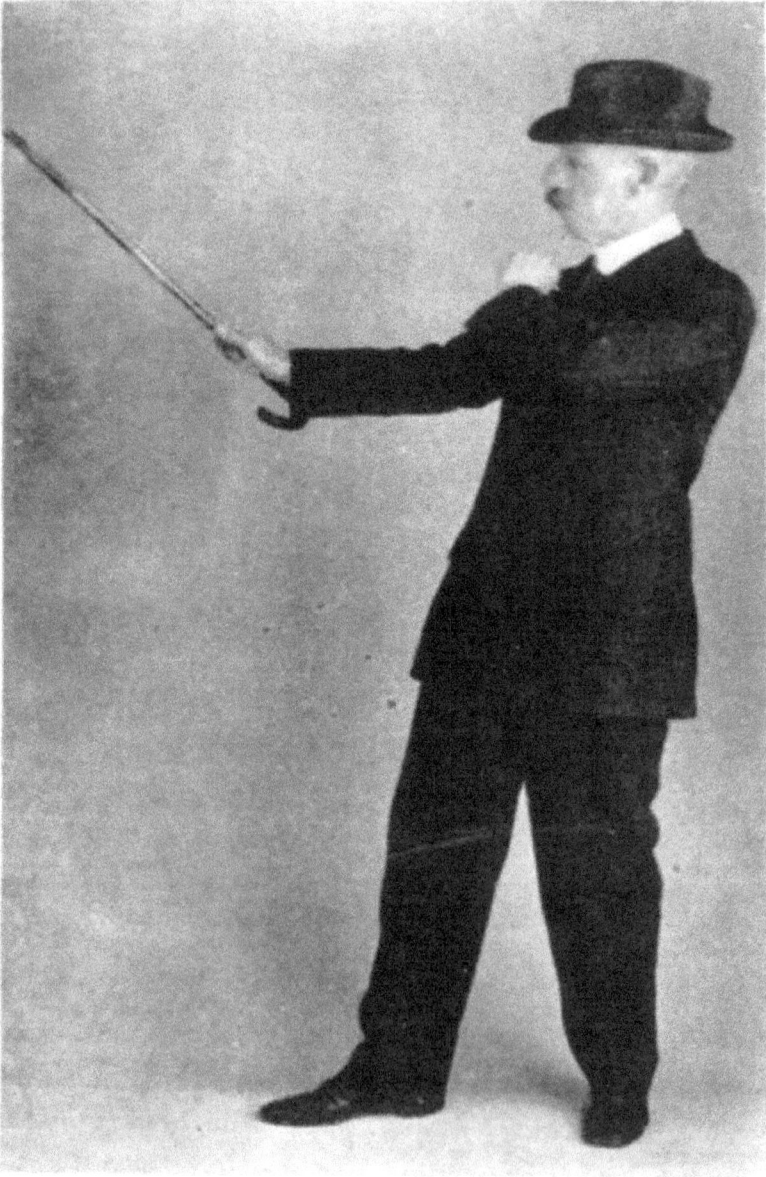

From right guard, right parry, high.

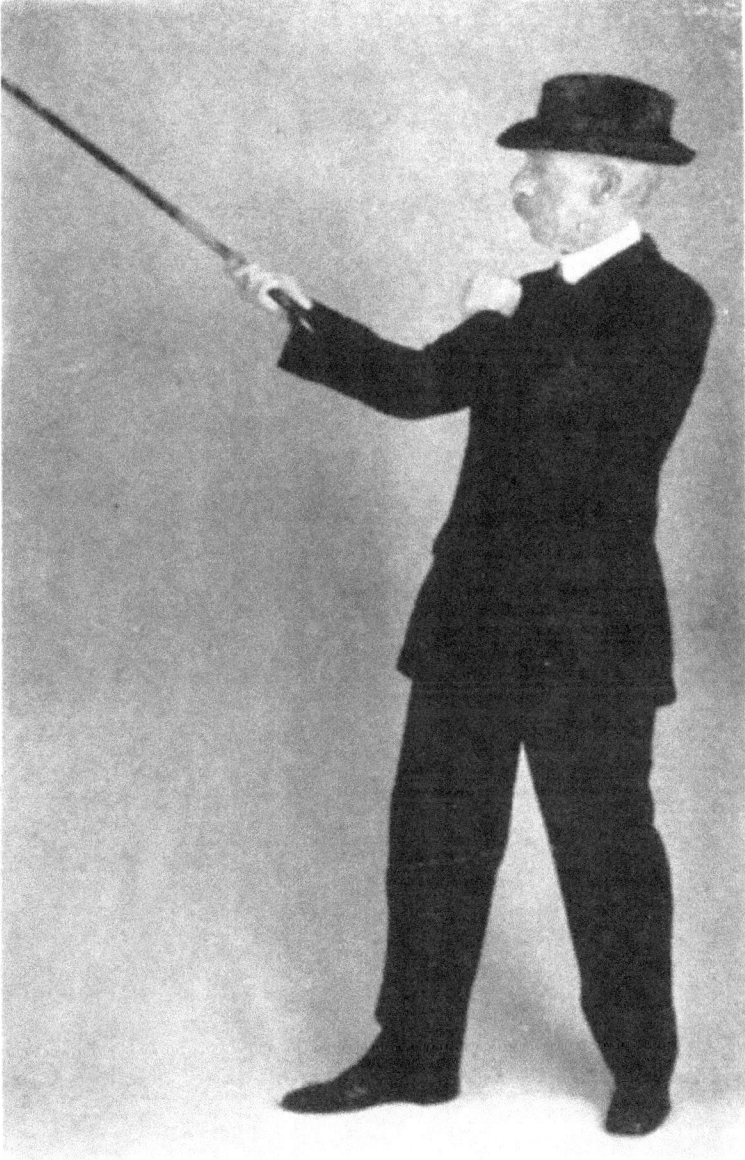

*From right guard, right counter parry after
adversary has parried left cut.*

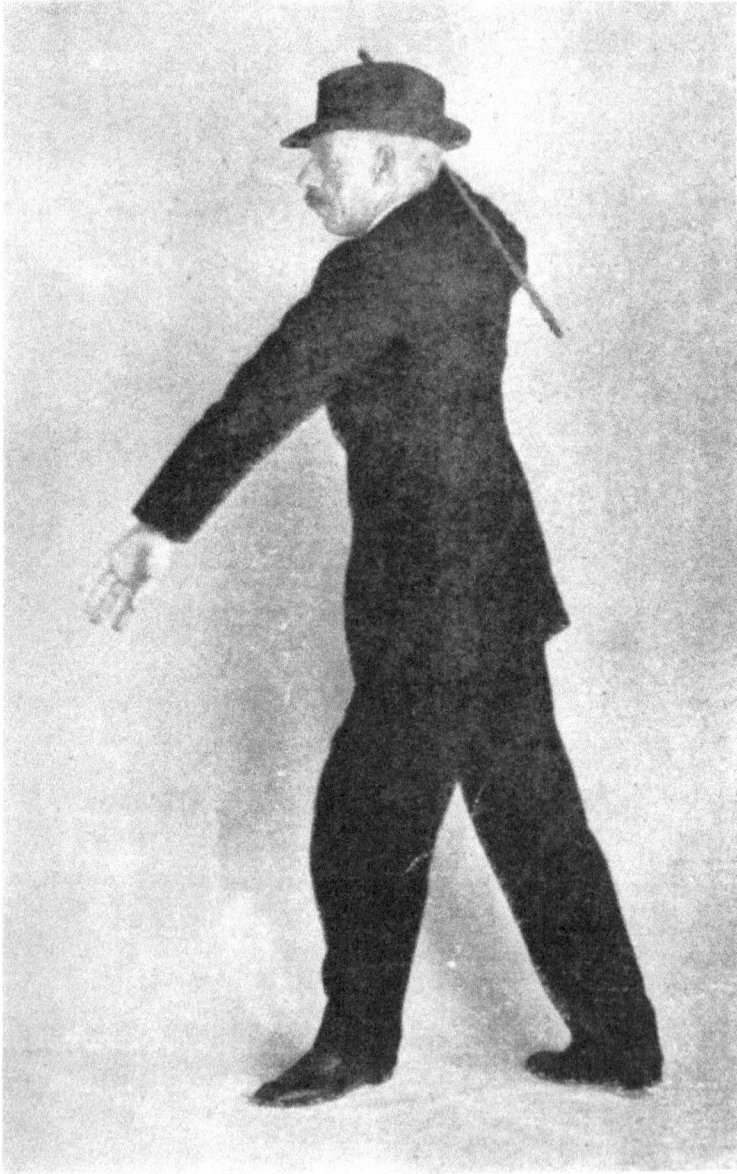

From right guard, rear pass half completed:
parry low thrust with left hand, and
full arm down cut to front.

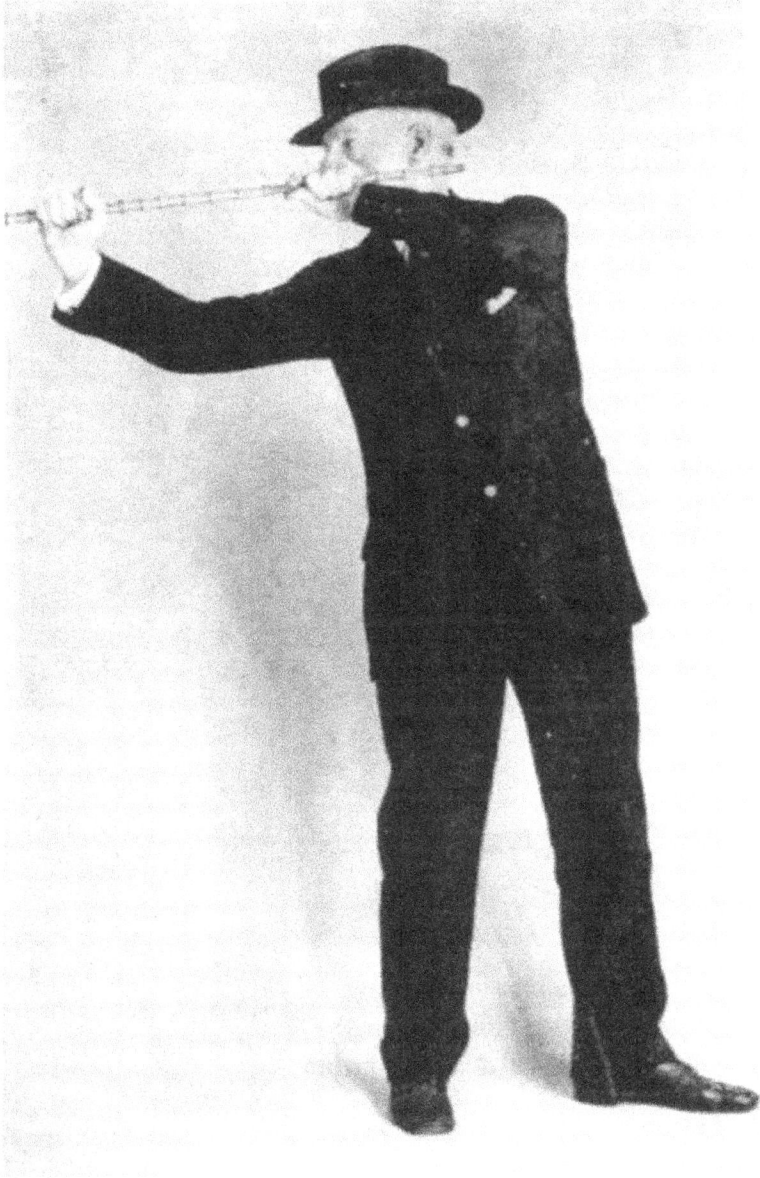

From double guard, left; jab high to
rear with butt.

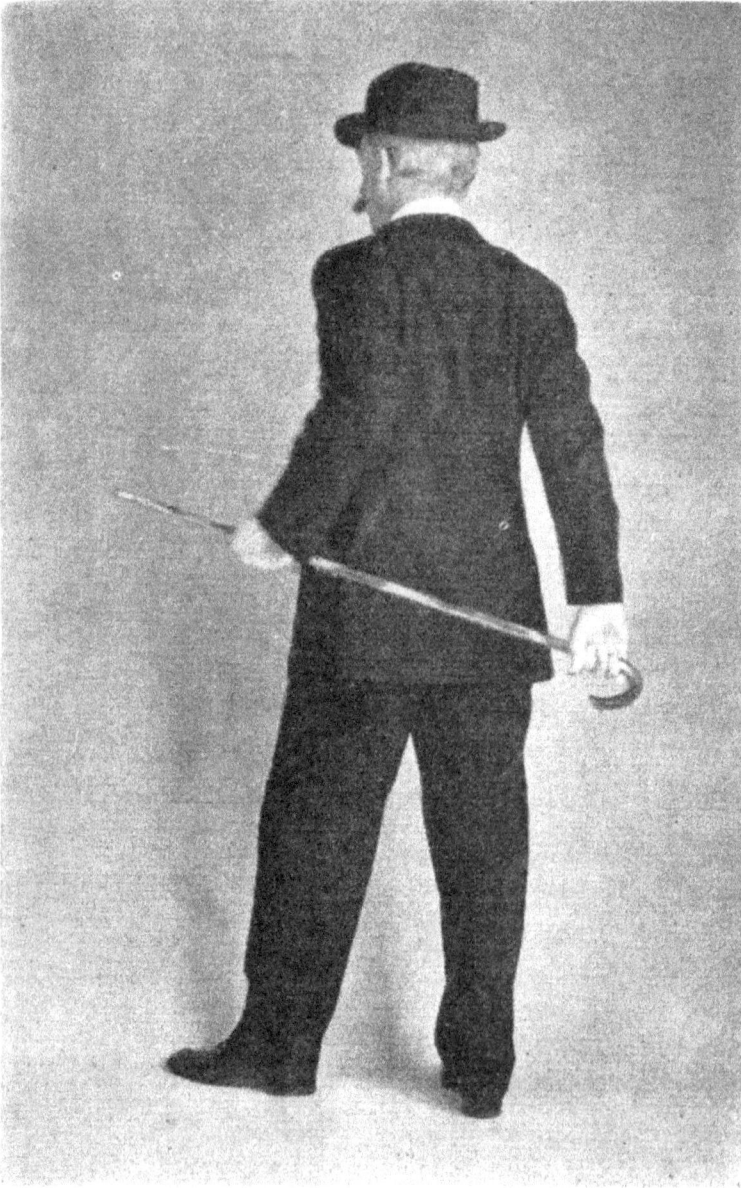

Off guard, grappled high in front; pass cane behind body to other hand and jab forward with point.

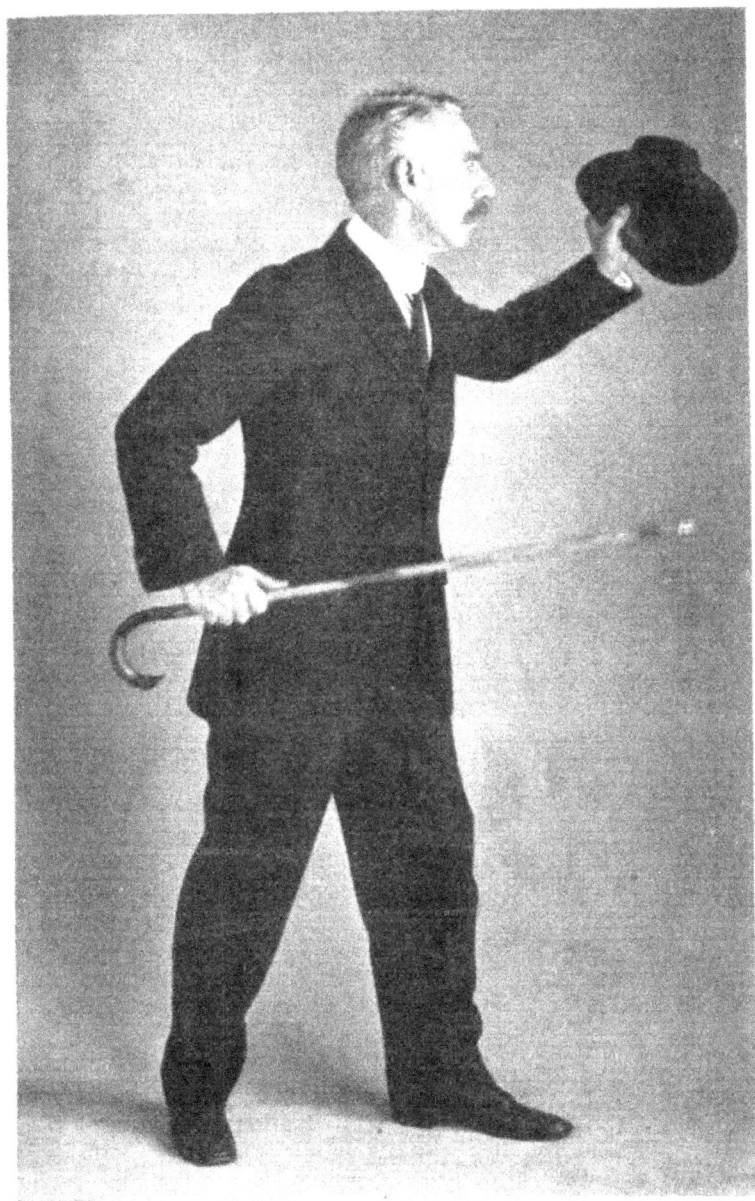

*From left guard; parry knife thrust with
the hat, and jab forward with point.*

www.ingramcontent.com/pod-product-compliance
Lightning Source LLC
Chambersburg PA
CBHW080609270326
41928CB00016B/2977